HIV&AIDS
KNOWLEDGE AND STIGMA IN GUYANA

HIV&AIDS
KNOWLEDGE AND STIGMA IN GUYANA

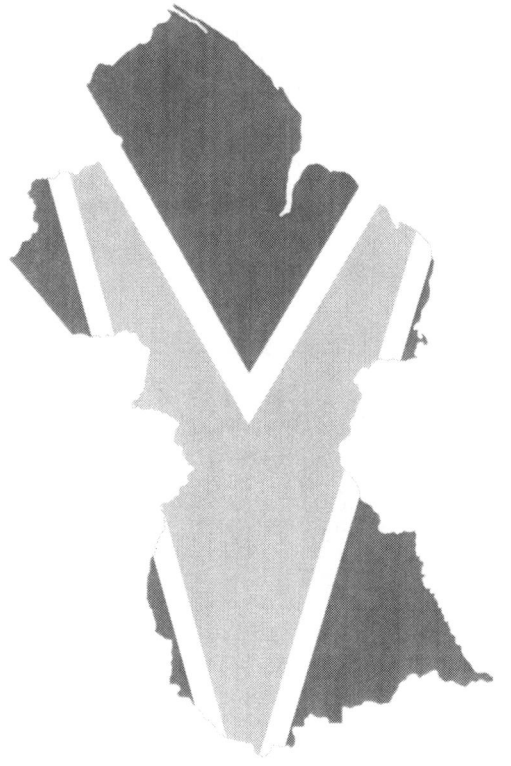

PREM MISIR

 THE UNIVERSITY OF THE WEST INDIES PRESS
Jamaica • Barbados • Trinidad and Tobago

The University of the West Indies Press
7A Gibraltar Hall Road, Mona
Kingston 7, Jamaica
www.uwipress.com

A catalogue record of this book is available from the National Library of Jamaica.

ISBN: 978-976-640-317-1 (paper)
ISBN: 978-976-640-417-8 (Kindle)
ISBN: 978-976-640-418-5 (ePub)

Cover design by Robert Harris
Production services: TIPS Technical Publishing, Inc.

Printed in the United States of America.

Contents

Figures

Tables

Foreword

"When you know better you do better."

– Maya Angelou

The first case of HIV in Guyana was reported in 1987. Presently, Guyana is described as having a generalized epidemic, and, if this trend continues, it will pose a threat to the social and economic development of the country.

While some headway is being made in the development of more effective HIV and AIDS treatment and resources are being channelled into various interventions, the level of stigma and discrimination related to HIV and AIDS is still a major issue. This acts as a barrier to the implementation of effective interventions in the fight against the diseases. HIV stigma is universal, but its form varies from country to country and the specific groups targeted vary considerably. Whatever its form, HIV stigma inflicts suffering on people and interferes with attempts to fight the epidemic. In 1988, the Institute of Medicine panel in the United States observed that "the fear of discrimination is a major constraint to the wide acceptance of many potentially effective public health measures".

Although widely recognized as a problem, HIV stigma has not been studied enough to inform policy makers and assist them to develop evidence-based, effective policies to fight the epidemic. This book, written by Professor Misir, goes a long way in bridging this gap by comprehensively studying HIV and AIDS knowledge and stigma among high school students in Guyana.

HIV, AIDS, and other diseases related to HIV and AIDS are the leading cause of death among the 20–49 age group in Guyana. Several of those with HIV or AIDS in their twenties would have contracted the infection in their adolescence. Limited understanding of the myths and misconceptions of HIV and AIDS in this group hampers the implementation of policies related to prevention, education and awareness. The premise of Professor Misir's research is that one of the main factors that determines who is stigmatized and why in Guyana will depend on the knowledge and beliefs of HIV and AIDS and it is therefore vital to understand the knowledge, myths and misconceptions. This will provide appropriate evidence-based information to policy makers to help them develop effective interventions to control the epidemic in Guyana.

The book sets the scene by outlining the picture of the present situation with HIV and AIDS in Guyana. It then goes on to study the literature related to knowledge and stigma-related attitudes/perceptions of HIV and AIDS. The comprehensive research undertaken to study Guyanese high school students' knowledge, attitudes/perceptions, and stigma-related attitudes/perceptions of HIV and AIDS and the implications of the findings is covered in detail. This book will make a major contribution to the development of evidence-based policy to fight the HIV and AIDS epidemic in Guyana and is a must read book for public health practitioners, researchers and students.

Charlotte Brontë wrote "prejudices, it is well known, are most difficult to eradicate from the heart whose soil has never been loosened or fertilized by education: they grow there, firm as weeds among stones". This book will both loosen and fertilize the soil in relation to the prejudice and stigma related to HIV and AIDS among young people in Guyana. It will contribute to ensuring that the weeds of stigma are uprooted and effective, and evidence-based prevention policies are implemented to support the response to the HIV and AIDS epidemic in Guyana.

Dr Premila Webster
MBBS, DA, MSc, MFPHM, FFPH,
DLATHE (Oxon), DPhil (Oxon)
Head of School of Public Health –
Oxford Deanery
Director of Education and Training,
Department of Public Health,
University of Oxford

Preface

No one would dispute the great damage that HIV and AIDS have inflicted on the global scene over the last three decades. Indeed, the harm remains phenomenal for poor societies where entire economies continue to experience devastation. As a former associate public health epidemiologist with the Bureau of HIV/AIDS Prevention and Control, New York City Department of Health and Mental Hygiene, I had the task as a principal investigator to respond to a Centers for Disease Control and Prevention grant request for studying the prevention of sexual transmission of HIV by HIV-seropositive men. This task enabled me to perceive the huge impact of stigma on people with HIV in the developed world, and its possible unparalleled damage on poor developing countries. And so my HIV and AIDS research vista on stigma at this juncture turned toward the global poor who are contracting HIV in their adolescent years.

This book arose out of my concerns over the likelihood of an increasing trend in high-risk sexual behaviours among adolescents in Guyana. These concerns relate to the perception that many adults in Guyana and elsewhere were graduating from HIV to an AIDS status in their twenties. Therefore, it is possible to conclude that many people with HIV in Guyana and elsewhere contracted the infection in their adolescence; hence, this study on HIV and AIDS knowledge and stigma among high school students in Guyana, of which this book is the short-term end product.

High school students were the unit of the study to compare differences in their HIV and AIDS knowledge and stigma-related attitudes. The study had a sample size of 379 African, Indian and mixed-race students aged thirteen to eighteen, with males and females, as well as Christians, Hindus and Muslims. The study attempted to answer these research questions:

- What is the status of HIV and AIDS knowledge and stigma-related attitudes/perceptions among high school students?
- What are the differences in HIV and AIDS knowledge and stigma-related attitudes by gender, age, religious groups and ethnic groups?

- Is there an overall relationship between HIV and AIDS knowledge and stigma-related attitudes?
- Is there a relationship between the non-normative aspects of HIV and AIDS knowledge and stigma-related attitudes?

Findings from this study will allow health professionals and educators to review the educational needs of high school students when it comes to understanding the basics of HIV and AIDS. The findings will enable health professionals and educators to appraise the sufficiency of high school students' knowledge of HIV and AIDS, how much knowledge of HIV and AIDS influences students' assimilation and application of stigma toward people living with HIV (PLHA), and the prerequisites for effective and efficient prevention intervention programmes.

Given the deficits in HIV preventive education among young people, the foremost distinguishing aspect of this study is that it targets adolescents within the 15 to 24 age group, who globally account for 40% of all new infections in adults. Another distinguishing aspect is that this study also concludes on the relationship between the non-normative aspects (misconceptions and myths) of HIV and AIDS knowledge and HIV and AIDS stigma.

During the research process, I started to realize the negative impact of misconceptions and myths of HIV and AIDS on high-risk sexual behaviours. Many prevention messages on stigma focus almost entirely on compliance with the conventional HIV and AIDS knowledge to the exclusion of misconceptions and myths, and thereby reducing the potency of the prevention message. I, however, would submit that prevention messages on stigma must incorporate both conventional HIV and AIDS knowledge as well as misconceptions and myths about HIV and AIDS.

An additional distinguishing aspect of this book is its presentation of the statistical procedures. This presentation provides some insights into the application of statistical procedures to enable the reader to become an informed user and consumer of statistics. I presented and validated assumptions for usage of each statistical procedure in order to show why I applied a particular procedure. I used descriptive statistics to measure the demographics and individual item scores on knowledge and attitudes; the independent samples t-test for differences between gender and knowledge, and age and knowledge; the Kruskal-Wallis (K-W) for differences among the religious persuasions and knowledge, and among ethnic groups and knowledge; independent samples t-test for differences between gender and stigma-related attitudes, and age and stigma-related attitudes; the ANOVA for differences among religious persuasions and stigma-related attitudes; the K-W for differences among ethnic groups and stigma-related attitudes; and the multiple logistic regression model to determine the variables influencing HIV and AIDS knowledge development and stigma-related attitudes toward HIV and AIDS.

There are seven chapters in this book. Chapter 1 is the introduction focusing on the response to HIV and AIDS, prevalence of HIV in Guyana, what we know of HIV and AIDS, deficiencies in research, significance of study, purpose of study, and research questions. Chapter 2 provides a review of the literature and a theoretical model of the literature. Chapter 3 covers the methodology of the study. Chapters 4, 5 and 6 offer the statistical analyses of the study: chapter 4 presents descriptive statistics on HIV and AIDS knowledge and demographics; chapter 5 addresses HIV and AIDS stigma-related attitudes/perceptions; and chapter 6 presents predictors of knowledge and stigma-related attitudes/perceptions. Chapter 7 puts forward the discussions and implications of the univariate, bivariate and multiple logistic regression findings of the study. The references also include recommended further readings, and I have included a large number of the tables in appendices by chapters.

My profound gratitude goes out to the Demerara Tobacco Company for its generous research award, a testimony to its commitment to fight HIV and AIDS among adolescents. I must convey considerable appreciation to the 379 students from fifteen high schools who participated in the field-work. These students will forever remain in my debt. I thank the Ministry of Education for the authorization to utilize high school students in the field work. Linda Speth of the University of the West Indies Press expressed great interest in this manuscript that helped me through the editing process. I would certainly like to thank the two anonymous reviewers of the University of the West Indies Press whose comprehensive and insightful comments were invaluable in refining the manuscript. I also appreciate the assistance of the University of the West Indies Press editorial and production team led by Shivaun Hearne. Finally, I feel privileged and honoured to have Dr Premila Webster of the Department of Public Health, University of Oxford, penning the foreword.

Chapter 1

Introduction

Three decades ago, a virus with major public health implications appeared. This virus, which continues to spread among the global population, is human immunodeficiency virus (HIV), of which acquired immunodeficiency syndrome (AIDS) can be the end-stage result. While there are precautionary measures one can take to avoid or limit one's chances of contracting this life-threatening virus, HIV remains a serious threat because the virus is transmittable as well as currently incurable.

Over the years, the number of recorded HIV cases and the number of AIDS-related deaths have remained high. In 2009, the United Nations Program on HIV and AIDS (UNAIDS) Global Report (2010) estimated that, worldwide, there were 33.3 million people living with HIV (PLHIV), compared to 26.2 million in 1999, showing a 27% increase. Of the 33.3 million PLHIV in 2009, 30.8 million were adults, 15.9 million were women and 2.5 million were children under age 15. In 2009, there were 2.6 million people newly infected with HIV compared to 3.1 million in 1999; in the same year, AIDS-related deaths totalled 1.8 million compared to 2.1 million recorded in 2004. Additionally, in 2009, about 370,000 children were newly infected with HIV, a decline of 24% from the previous five years.

UNAIDS Global Report (2010) estimated the regional adult HIV prevalence in 2009 as shown in table 1.1.

In 2009, UNAIDS presented nine priorities for addressing the HIV pandemic. UNAIDS viewed the purpose of these priorities as a way to direct investment and marshal resources for focused and intensive action.

Table 1.1 Regional Adult HIV Prevalence, 2009

Region	Per Cent Total
Sub-Saharan Africa	5.0
Middle East & North Africa	0.2
South and South-East Asia	0.3
East Asia	0.1
Central & South America	0.5
Oceania	0.3
Caribbean	1.0
Eastern Europe & Central Asia	0.8
Western & Central Europe	0.2
North America	0.5
Total	0.8

Source: UNAIDS Report on the Global AIDS Epidemic, 2010

Outlined below is the UNAIDS Outcome Framework (2009–2011) of the nine priority areas:

1. We can reduce sexual transmission of HIV.
2. We can prevent mothers from dying and babies from becoming infected with HIV.
3. We can ensure that people living with HIV receive treatment.
4. We can prevent people living with HIV from dying of tuberculosis.
5. We can protect drug users from becoming infected with HIV.
6. We can remove punitive laws, policies, practices, stigma and discrimination that block effective responses to HIV.
7. We can stop violence against women and girls.
8. We can empower young people to protect themselves from HIV.
9. We can enhance social protection for people affected by HIV.

   Guyana has begun to address several of these priorities, such as the Prevention of Mother-to-Child-Transmission (PMTCT). In 2010, there were 165 PMTCT sites nationally, and these sites offer programmes to prevent HIV infection from mother to child during pregnancy, labour and delivery, or breast feeding. Fathers will soon constitute a vital part of the PMTCT programme.

Response to HIV and AIDS

To acquire a better understanding of the AIDS epidemic in Guyana, readers need to be acquainted with a few facts. To begin with, Guyana, with a population of 751,223, had its first ten cases of AIDS in 1987, and the incidence of infection rose in subsequent years. In the late 1980s, Guyana had a limited capacity to address the evolving epidemic, and during the same period, the Caribbean Epidemiology Centre (CAREC) agreed to receive samples of suspected cases for testing.

The consistent increasing incidence of HIV cases in the late 1980s demanded the establishment of a national programme and response. Consequently, a National AIDS Committee entered the scene in 1989 to counsel the Ministry of Health on the possibility of developing a national HIV and AIDS programme. In 1992, the government created the National AIDS Programme Secretariat (NAPS) to manage the epidemic, with particular emphasis on the risk factors. Afterward, CAREC, the European Commission and the Pan American Health Organization/World Health Organization (PAHO/WHO) supported the setting up of the Genito-Urinary Medicine (GUM) Clinic, the National Laboratory for Infectious Disease (NLID) and the National Blood Transfusion Service (NBTS).

As a response to the HIV epidemic in the Caribbean, the Caribbean HIV and AIDS Task Force, created by the Caribbean Community (CARICOM) in 1998, presented a Caribbean Regional Strategic Plan for HIV and AIDS 2002–2006. The strategic plan was designed to lend support to emergent national programmes within the structure of the Pan Caribbean Partnership (PANCAP). International and regional developments also spurred the Caribbean response. The United Nations General Assembly Special Session (UNGASS), for instance, sanctioned the need to reduce HIV prevalence among the 15–24 age group of both males and females. The assembly also affirmed the need to incorporate prevention interventions at the workplace and to implement universal infection control procedures. At the Twenty-sixth Special Session of the UNGASS, support was given to the following resolution:

> By 2003, establish time bound national targets to achieve the internationally agreed prevention goal to reduce by 2005 HIV prevalence among young men and women aged 15–24 in the most affected countries by 25% and by 25% globally by 2010, and intensify efforts to achieve these targets as well as to challenge gender stereotypes and attitudes and gender inequalities in relation to HIV/AIDS, encouraging the active involvement of men and boys; by 2005, strengthen the response to HIV/AIDS in the world of work by establishing and implementing prevention and care programmes in public, private and informal work sectors and take

measures to provide a supportive workplace environment for people living with HIV/AIDS. . . . By 2003, implement universal precautions in health-care settings to prevent transmission of HIV infection.

The Nassau Declaration at the end of the CARICOM Heads of Government Meeting in 2001 recognized the overwhelming impact of HIV and AIDS on the young in their most productive years. Heads pledged support for the UNGASS statement, adopted a consolidated approach to utilize benefits from the UN Global HIV and AIDS Health Fund and continued to support PANCAP. It is useful to mention these regional and international developments because they drive national governments' responses to HIV and AIDS, including those of Guyana.

In Guyana, in the late 1980s and a greater part of the 1990s, there was no strategic plan to address the HIV issue; the first National Strategic Plan for HIV was presented as late as 1999–2001. The second National Strategic Plan, 2002–2006, focused on crafting an enabling environment for an appropriate national workplace. Additionally, the plan proposed legislation on non-discrimination against PLHIV, supported the provision of HIV funding in at least five government ministries and endorsed the revision of public health laws pertaining to infectious diseases. Subsequently, the Ministry of Health operationalized the National HIV Strategy, 2007–2011.

The UNAIDS already is on record as indicating that Guyana may be experiencing one of the most severe epidemics in Latin America and the Caribbean. In the early years of the HIV infection in Guyana, the workplace was not considered a site for distributing information and education on HIV. For one thing, the workplace as an information site was new. Furthermore, no urgency was attributed to the virus within the business community, so there were limited awareness and advocacy campaigns. Today, both UNGASS and CARICOM acknowledge the potential for high-risk behaviours and the predominance of out-of-school young people in the 15–24 age group, both of which are factors that make the workplace a significant target for reducing HIV transmission.

NAPS in 2000 disseminated to several work sites a brochure titled "HIV and the Workplace" (2000). The brochure focused on three areas: producing a workplace policy, negotiating employee human resource benefits and developing a workplace programme. However, the brochure elicited a limited national workplace response. The Information, Education and Communication (IEC) programme at NAPS and the Occupational Safety and Health (OSH) Department of the Ministry of Labour initiated sensitization programmes on HIV at the workplace for both public and private enterprises. In 2001, Occupational Safety and Health Officers from the Ministry of Labour, Barama, Linmine, the Guyana Sugar Corporation (GuySuCo), the Mayor and City Council (M&CC), the Georgetown Sewerage and Water Commissioners (GS&WC), the Guyana National Industrial Company (GNIC), Banks D'Aguiar Imperial Holdings (DIH), and the Guyana National Shipping Corporation (GNSC) received training in HIV and AIDS awareness. This initiative resulted in approximately six hundred workplaces administering awareness and education sessions to about fourteen thousand workers. In fact, most workplace responses over the last five years were mainly intermittent sensitization and awareness sessions directed at workers.

GuySuCo is one of the few corporations making significant strides in what in other respects is commonly an indifferent national response to HIV at the workplace. GuySuCo's workplace policy includes training for health workers in managing PLHIV, confidential pre- and post-test counselling and no mandatory testing as a pre-condition for employment. Following closely in GuySuCo's stride is the Georgetown Public Hospital Corporation (GPHC) which has established a committee to monitor the implementation of its workplace HIV policy.

A subcommittee of the National Tripartite Committee was expected to formulate HIV workplace policies for subsequent infusion in collective labour agreements and occupational safety and health regimes which are still awaiting institutionalization. The subcommittee has representatives from the Ministry of Labour, the Consultative Association of Guyanese Industry and the Guyana Trades Union Congress.

The establishment of the Presidential Panel on HIV and AIDS (PPHA) in January 2004 has become a significant catalyst to establishing workplace HIV and AIDS policies and programmes. The PPHA has prompted the establishment of ministerial committees mandated to produce workplace HIV policies in various ministries. World Bank funding of US$10M was allocated to this project.

Prevalence of HIV in Guyana

The largest number of HIV cases has been reported among the 15–49 age groups (table 1.2). This group largely comprises the workforce of 271,728 persons, 69% of whom are males and 31% of whom are females (Census Road 2002). Figure 1.1 shows that between 1991 and 2001, an average of 58% of the national workforce aged 20 to 39 accounted for about 68% of the reported HIV cases.

HIV has affected the lives of workers in Guyana, ranging from senior managers to lower skilled workers. Table 1.3 indicates that the largest number of AIDS cases is among low-skilled and service workers, such as sales workers, technicians, craft and trade workers, minibus operators, and general elementary workers. Considering that the disease predominantly

Table 1.2 Distribution of HIV Cases by Age Group, 2009

Age Groups	Total	Distribution by Age Group
<1 yr	1	0.08
1–4	9	0.76
5–4	14	1.19
15–19	71	6.03
20–24	136	11.56
25–29	161	13.69
30–34	204	17.34
35–39	198	16.83
40–44	143	12.15
45–49	105	8.92
50–54	48	4.08
55–59	30	2.55
60+	25	2.12
Unknown	21	2.63
Total	1,176	100.0%

Source: Ministry of Health Statistics Unit

Table 1.3 Distribution of AIDS Cases by Age Group, 2009

Age Groups	Total	Distribution by Age Group
5–14	1	2.32
15–19	1	2.32
20–24	7	16.27
25–29	4	9.3
30–34	5	11.62
35–39	8	18.6
40–44	6	13.95
45–49	6	13.95
50–54	3	6.97
55–59	1	2.32
Unknown	1	2.32
Total	43	100.0%

Source: Ministry of Health Statistics Unit

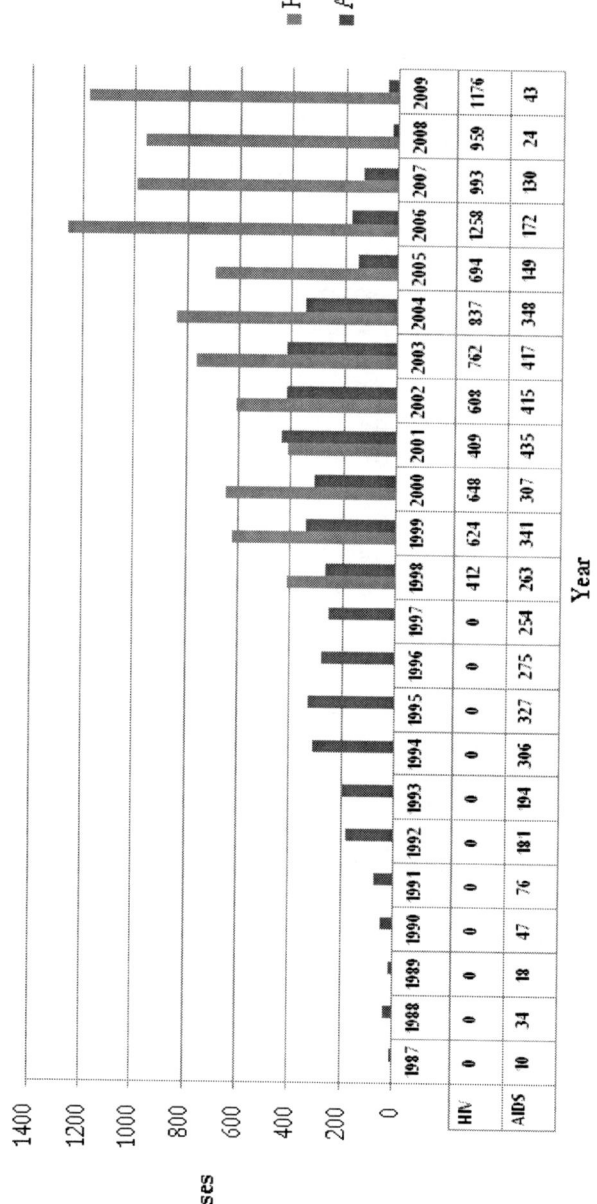

	1987	1988	1989	1990	1991	1992	1993	1994	1995	1996	1997	1998	1999	2000	2001	2002	2003	2004	2005	2006	2007	2008	2009
HIV	0	0	0	0	0	0	0	0	0	0	0	412	624	648	409	608	762	837	694	1258	993	959	1176
AIDS	10	34	18	47	76	181	194	306	327	275	254	263	341	307	435	415	417	348	149	172	130	24	43

Figure 1.1 Prevalence of HIV and AIDS in Guyana, 1987–2009
Source: Ministry of Health Statistics Unit

afflicts the young, one can reasonably assume that the quality and quantity of the workforce can be negatively affected. Among other outcomes, HIV can compromise the economy and increase rates of family disintegration and the number of children orphaned due to AIDS.

It is important to point out that during the initial phases of the HIV outbreak in Guyana, information and education about HIV was not distributed in the workplace. Interestingly, for the years 1999 and 2001, 58% of the labour force aged 20 to 39 represented about 50% of the reported HIV cases. If the possible progression of the HIV infection to the onset of AIDS occurs between a year or less and ten years or more, then a large number of AIDS-infected persons in their twenties would have contracted HIV in their adolescence (Imperato 1996).

Hancock et al. (1999) noted that a major concern is the heterosexual transmission of HIV among adolescents. They noted, too, that developmentally, adolescents are generally at high risk for contracting the HIV infection. Walker (1992) believes that adolescence represents a period involving high-risk behaviours, such as sexual activities and experimentation with illicit drugs. Clearly, high-risk behaviours can increase the incidence of HIV contraction. For this reason, it is critical that we continuously engage in studies that assess adolescents' knowledge of HIV and AIDS as well as adolescents' at-risk behaviours.

Based on the information provided by the Ministry of Health Statistics Unit, one can conclude that the number of HIV cases recorded from 1998 to 2009 was significantly high, particularly in the years 2006 to 2009, with 2006 recording the highest number of HIV cases (1,258) and 2009 recording the second highest (1,176 cases). Similarly, the number of AIDS cases recorded was very high, specifically during the years 1994 to 2004. However, during the years 2005 to 2009, the number of AIDS cases sharply declined, with the most significant decrease recorded in 2008 (24 cases). In effect, figure 1.1 shows a steady increase in the prevalence of HIV since 2003, but a steady decline in AIDS cases since 2006. This consistently high HIV prevalence and low AIDS prevalence indicate that PLHIV have a higher survival rate, largely the result of the availability of, accessibility to and effectiveness of antiretroviral treatment.

In 2009, eighty-five (18%) HIV cases were recorded from the 5–14 and 15–19 age groups, and only two (5%) cases reached the onset of AIDS. Currently, there are an increasing number of HIV cases among adolescents which could produce another increase in AIDS cases. These statistics represent important justifications for a study on HIV and AIDS knowledge and stigma-related attitudes/perceptions of adolescent high school students.

Since the advent of multiple-source funding from the Global AIDS Fund, the US President's Emergency Plan for AIDS Relief (PEPFAR), UNICEF and the World Bank, the Guyana response to combating HIV through its non-governmental organizations (NGOs) and public health sector remains an urgent policy-of-choice. Ranging from abstinence to condom usage for both males and females, these policies constitute the centre of a passionate national debate. The religious bodies, for example, use theology to stir the debate on appropriate interventions in the responses to HIV and AIDS.

Guyana continues to advance its prevention programme services to key and high-risk populations, instituting over 165 Prevention of Mother-to-Child-Transmission sites by 2010. It is also timely that PEPFAR has begun to reallocate resources from direct service delivery to capacity building for both workers and the at-risk populations, for it would hardly be an overemphasis to underline the importance of HIV and AIDS knowledge for both groups.

Guyana, with a high prevalence of HIV in the Caribbean, has a dearth of scientific studies addressing the awareness, behaviours and probable points of entry for HIV contraction. Also, with the maturity of the disease, more people are contracting it at a young age. This means, therefore, that HIV affects people in their prime of life, with possible negative repercussions for education and work productivity.

What We Know of HIV and AIDS

At the end of the fourth decade of the HIV epidemic, there still is no cure, so our method of minimizing HIV has to be seeking behavioural changes, public education and complying with universal precautions. UNESCO's Gudmund Hermes (2001) remarked about AIDS, thus: "The virus was ahead of the disease, the disease was ahead of the response, the response was a disaster, and management of the disaster was underfunded." Today, with greater funding, the response is still inadequate through skill incapacity and bureaucratic constraints.

Additionally, the HIV field today has become highly opinionated with people jockeying to present inputs to address the epidemic, a good in itself, nevertheless, inputs that must be subject to assessment, monitoring and evaluation, and inputs that comply with the standards of the scientific community that has determined the following to be true:

- an increasing number of Guyanese are directly and indirectly impacted by the HIV infection and AIDS, the impact touching each population segment and geographical location of this country;
- people in their prime of life are the most affected by HIV and AIDS;
- as the epidemic becomes matured, people contract the HIV infection at a young age;
- women are at higher risk from heterosexual transmission than men;
- with the current higher maturity level of the disease, the infection is transmitted from the initial high-risk groups into the larger society;

- the HIV epidemic will impact every workplace with protracted staff illness, absenteeism and death – all of which will have serious repercussions on productivity, employee benefits, occupational health and safety, and costs of production;
- that the most helpful way of reducing and managing HIV effects at the workplace is through the development and implementation of an HIV policy programme;
- the HIV infection that causes AIDS is transmitted from person to person only in specific ways, and not through casual contact;
- no known cure currently exists, but existing antiretroviral treatments delay disease progression, making HIV a manageable chronic disease;
- behaviour changes, public education and universal precautions are the best practices in prevention intervention;
- HIV is an infectious disease, and that infectious diseases including those related to HIV prevail at the workplace;
- the virus does not survive outside the human body;
- despite the increase in technical knowledge of HIV, there still is rapid transmission;
- HIV and AIDS-related stigma and discrimination are huge barriers to prevention efforts.

In 2001, the Commission on Macroeconomics and Health (CMH), a unit of the WHO, branded the HIV epidemic as an unparalleled crisis that needs special consideration. The CMH concluded that twenty years into the epidemic, millions of young people still have minimum knowledge of HIV and AIDS as well as critical misconceptions about how HIV is transmitted.

Deficiencies in Research

Some deficiencies in research prevail in the following areas:
   Adults (19–60 years)

- On more information pertaining to the cure and transmission of HIV
- On innovative and culturally sensitive sexual and reproductive health programmes to change at-risk sexual behaviour
- On public policy addressing discriminatory responses
- On minimizing misconceptions about HIV transmission
- On the use of a family-based approach to reduce transmission of HIV and to increase knowledge of HIV and AIDS
- On interventions promoting greater interaction of PLHIV and non-infected persons vis-à-vis reducing stigma
- On the main reasons for HIV transmission
- On marshalling the religious forces to reduce enactment of stigma toward PLHIV

Adolescents (13–18 years)

- On the culture of the people when instituting HIV intervention programmes
- On more interventions on attitude change
- On greater interaction among PLHIV and adolescents to minimize negative attitudes/perceptions
- On males requiring effective education programmes
- On cultural difficulties, such as where a culture dissuades discussions of sexuality
- On females in a male-dominated society
- On more HIV education for minority groups
- On areas of misunderstanding and prevention interventions
- On younger age groups requiring a better skill-set to address HIV and AIDS
- On parental involvement in HIV and AIDS education
- On dysfunctional families without the wherewithal to provide HIV education
- On health providers without the skill-set to communicate with adolescents
- On religious and conservative groups' opposition to gender education in schools
- On educating adolescents in rural areas

The HIV population has matured indicating that people are contracting the HIV infection at a younger age. This situation, in which at-risk heterosexual activity is the main mode of HIV transmission, would suggest that adolescents are quite sexually active. For this reason, we need to find out how much young people know about HIV and AIDS and what their attitudes/perceptions are of PLHIV. This information would be fundamental in our efforts to develop effective interventions to reduce the spread of HIV transmission. When one considers that two-thirds of Guyana's population is 35 years and under; that the active working population is between ages 16 and 55; and that between 1999 and 2001, 58% of the national workforce aged 20 to 39 comprised about 50% of the reported HIV cases, one would understand the urgent need for school education programmes as well as a comprehensive national HIV and AIDS workplace policy.

Significance of Study

School-based HIV prevention intervention programmes have a significant role to play in HIV prevention in Guyana. With about half (50.9%) of Guyana's population under age 24 and about 70% under age 14 (Population and Housing Census 2002), schools have an in-built infrastructure with extensive reach during a crucial developmental period (Yazdi et al. 2006). Adolescents are also appropriate targets for school-based interventions because their attitudes and behaviours are still being developed (NIH 1997; UNAIDS/WHO 2004). Interventions have a higher success rate when introduced before the target group begins experimentation with risk behaviours (Grunseit 1997). For these reasons, this study in reviewing baseline HIV and AIDS knowledge levels and stigma-related attitudes among adolescents in Guyana presents a vital foundation for appropriate prevention intervention programmes.

Since the progression of the HIV infection to the possible onset of AIDS can occur between a year or less and ten years or more, a large number of AIDS-infected persons in their twenties would have contracted the infection in their adolescence. In Guyana, in 2009, there were 71 (6.03%) cases in the 15–19 age group with HIV, and 1 case (2.32%) in the 15–19 age group with AIDS (UNGASS 2010). Given that Guyana has a national population of less than three-quarters of a million people and that such HIV and AIDS statistics among young people exists, there is, indeed, justification for this study on HIV and AIDS knowledge and HIV and AIDS stigma-related attitudes/perceptions among adolescents in high schools.

In addition, the Caribbean has the highest HIV prevalence, excepting sub-Saharan Africa, with the highest prevalence in men having sex with men (MSM) and sex workers (SW). Young people who are also MSM or SW or both represent the most highly affected communities (MARPS) (UNGASS 2004, 2006, 2008). Inciardi, Syvertsen and Surratt (2005) indicated that sexual transmission of HIV is enhanced through early initiation of sexual intercourse, having multiple partners and older men having sexual intercourse with young girls in the Caribbean; these practices significantly increase the HIV infection rate among young people. In addition, about 50% of new HIV infections occur among young people aged 15 to 24 in Latin America and the Caribbean (PAHO 2003). In CAREC Centre member countries, young women aged 15 to 24 are more significantly infected, where the annual HIV incidence rate is three to six times greater than males within the same age range (Camara et al. 2003). The UNAIDS report on the Caribbean (2010) suggested that young people are amenable to change, and attempts made to inculcate appropriate knowledge, attitudes, beliefs on HIV and AIDS, and sexually transmitted infections (STIs) may help to prevent HIV transmission.

Kelly and Bain (2004) noted that the first two decades of the HIV epidemic in the Caribbean embraced responses mainly confined to the health sector, and only now is there a response from the education sector. At the launch of the Campaign on Advocacy and Leadership to Advance the Caribbean Education Sector Response to HIV and AIDS (2005), Whitman explained that "It is crucial to move beyond tradition – beyond the tradition of the education sector's focus primarily on academics and beyond the tradition of a curriculum-only approach to HIV/AIDS. The education sector's influence in society is crucial in saving generations of Caribbean youth as it leads in countering stigma and discrimination and a deepened response for teachers and students."

As the education sector's response attempts to impact HIV, young people in the Caribbean are at high risk of contracting HIV; just note the following: "Of the one-third who are sexually active, half report that sexual intercourse was forced and half of the boys and about one quarter of the girls say that their age of first intercourse was ten years old. Almost two-thirds had intercourse before the age of 13. Males were about three times more likely than females to have five or more sexual partners" (Halcon, Beuhring and Blum 2000, 14). With this one-third not using condoms, they are a key population particularly vulnerable to HIV infection (UNAIDS 2011). Furthermore, given there is a continuous increase in HIV contraction rates among Caribbean women and the fact that they probably feature in among the highest cervical cancer rates globally, which has a connection with STIs (PAHO 2003), then there is a serious need for schools to respond to children quite early. Therefore, this is more justification for this study on HIV and AIDS knowledge and HIV and AIDS stigma-related attitudes/perceptions among a sample of high school students in Guyana. In addition, it is now well established that stigma is a formidable barrier that prevents any effective control of HIV. It is also well established that knowledge of HIV and AIDS has a mixed impact on individuals' attitudes/perceptions of the disease (Manji, Pena and Dubrow 2007; Dias et al. 2006; Hongjie et al. 2006; Lau, Tsui and Chan 2005; Tavoosi et al. 2004). Most studies conducted to ascertain individuals' knowledge of HIV have focused on the normative aspects of the disease, that is, on its modes of transmission, and this approach may not be enough to make definitive conclusions on the overall state and impact of HIV and AIDS knowledge, stigma-related attitudes/perceptions and stigma-reduction intervention designs. This study is significant, too, because it seeks to determine the relationship between the non-normative aspects (myths and misconceptions) of HIV and AIDS knowledge and stigma-related attitudes/perceptions.

Purpose of Study

Given that there are serious deficiencies in comprehensive HIV preventive education among young people, the major distinguishing feature of this study is that it targets a national sample of high school students aged 13 to 18. While there is no data on the infection rate among high school students in Guyana, their age range falling within the 15 to 24 age group is critical in that 40% of all new infections in adults worldwide are within the 15 to 24 age group.

The purpose of this study stems from the premise that stigmatizing attitudes and beliefs negatively impact interventions to prevent and treat HIV and AIDS, and since one of the basic factors that may determine stigmatizing attitudes and beliefs is a lack of knowledge of the disease, it is critical to establish what the level of this knowledge is in Guyana. Therefore, the purpose of this study was to test the relationship between high school students' HIV and AIDS knowledge and their stigma-related attitudes/perceptions of PLHIV. HIV and AIDS knowledge was divided into impact of the disease; symptoms; myths and misconceptions of HIV transmission; clinical modes of HIV transmission; HIV testing; blood donation; and preventative measures. The second part of this study asked the student participants to identify their stigma-related attitudes toward PLHIV and HIV and AIDS. Stigma-related attitudes were defined by perceptions of HIV and AIDS as death; perceptions of HIV and AIDS as punishment; perceptions of HIV and AIDS as crime; perceptions of HIV and AIDS as horror; perceptions of being insusceptible to HIV and AIDS; perceptions of HIV and AIDS as derision; perceptions of HIV and AIDS as social exclusion and marginalization; and perceptions of HIV and AIDS as social labelling and stereotyping.

Research Questions

The research seeks to address the following questions:

- What is the status of HIV and AIDS knowledge and stigma-related attitudes/perceptions among high school students?
- What are the differences in HIV and AIDS knowledge and stigma-related attitudes/perceptions by demographic variables of gender, age, religious groups and ethnicity?
- Is there an overall relationship between HIV and AIDS knowledge and stigma-related attitudes/perceptions?
- Is there a relationship between the non-normative aspects of HIV and AIDS knowledge and stigma-related attitudes/perceptions?

Chapter 2

Literature Review

HIV and AIDS Knowledge and Stigma-related Attitudes/Perceptions

To answer the research questions pertaining to HIV and AIDS knowledge and stigma-related attitudes/perceptions among high school students, the Population Intervention Comparison Outcome (PICO) search strategy was used to elicit answers on "HIV or AIDS and knowledge and stigma-related attitudes/perceptions". Electronic databases of Medline and PsycInfo were employed, hand searches were conducted and reference lists of articles retrieved were reviewed for citation purposes to maximize the researcher's capacity to identify appropriate articles focusing on HIV preventive education among young people. There was no time restriction on the search.

The UNAIDS (2010) noted serious deficiencies in comprehensive HIV preventive education among young people, even though 40% of all new infections in adults are among young people aged 15 to 24, the age group at the greatest risk for HIV infection. Studies over two decades have shown that for every five people living with AIDS, one person is between 20 and 29 years old (CDC 1993; Smith et al. 1993), and due to the long HIV incubation phase, the possibility exists that older adolescents and younger adults living with AIDS in their twenties probably would have contracted the HIV infection as young teenagers (Stall, Coates and Hoff 1988; Curran et al. 1988; Gordon et al. 2012; Kennedy and Jenkins 2011). Sechrist (1997) purported that initial sexual experiences, large prevalence of STIs and addiction are factors that place young people at a higher risk of HIV infection, and that in the absence of a cure or vaccine for HIV, the viable option available is prevention.

Numerous studies show that contracting HIV is preventable through behavioural interventions vis-à-vis developing HIV and AIDS knowledge on prevention, transmission, treatment and care, and that it is critical to reduce stigma-related attitudes/perceptions of PLHIV since stigma is a major barrier to prevention efforts. For these reasons, the purpose of this literature review is to assess high school students' knowledge of HIV and AIDS as well as these students' attitudes and perceptions toward PLHIV with the view to design effective behavioural prevention intervention programmes.

Välimäki, Suominen and Peate (1998) provided a holistic review of the literature on attitudes towards HIV and AIDS and PLHIV in the 1990s. This study reviewed the research on the attitudes of healthcare professionals, students and the general public to HIV and AIDS and PLHIV. Most of the studies covered the United States, United Kingdom, Australia, Canada, China, Denmark, Germany, France, Hungary, Israel, Italy, Kenya, the Netherlands, New Zealand, Norway, Portugal, Tanzania, Uganda and Zimbabwe. They all portrayed the fears, misconceptions and negative attitudes that people have toward HIV and AIDS and PLHIV. The review of findings in this study emphasized four dimensions: (1) research interest in HIV and AIDS attitudes grew in the 1990s; (2) most of the studies were empirical research conducted in the US; (3) the studies focused on students and their attitudes toward HIV and AIDS and sexual behaviour; and (4) the questionnaire design was the most popular method of data gathering.

Välimäki, Suominen and Peate (1998) also found that knowledge had a connection with fears and misconceptions, and therefore it was important to increase knowledge of HIV and AIDS. Since their study demonstrated that education had a differential impact on different groups, the search for the most appropriate teaching methods was necessary. The review also found that experiences shaped attitudes, and that the most positive attitudes had associations with caring for PLHIV.

HIV and AIDS Knowledge

Sallar (2009) found that over twenty-five years into the HIV pandemic, there was still a high level of misconceptions about HIV and AIDS. Sallar conducted a cross-sectional quantitative and qualitative study of 483 adolescents aged 10 to 19 in the Ashanti region in Ghana to determine their HIV and AIDS knowledge, misconceptions and attitudes toward PLHIV. The adolescents had good knowledge of HIV and AIDS in terms of sexual abstinence, condom use, fidelity to partner, not sharing needles and reducing sexual partners. But there were misconceptions: some students heard that medical doctors, herbalists/traditional healers and spiritualists could produce a cure for AIDS; there was the belief among some students that fate was the determinant as to whether or not a person contracts HIV; and there were those students who believed that they would not become ill, regardless of their actions.

A study of Flemish high school students drawn from eighty-five randomly selected schools in Flanders (Rossem, Berten and Tuyckom 2010) showed that those with high socioeconomic status had good knowledge of HIV and AIDS, and the reverse situation occurred for those with low socioeconomic status; moreover, females had better knowledge of HIV and AIDS than males, and fifth graders demonstrated better knowledge than third graders, suggesting that knowledge of HIV and AIDS increased with age.

Agius et al. (2010) conducted a study in Australia on sexual health knowledge and risk behaviours among secondary school students aged 13 to 18 between 1997 and 2008. They sampled students from 300 schools from the government, independent and Catholic school sectors. Both male and female students showed good knowledge of HIV and AIDS, and year 12 students had better knowledge of HIV and AIDS than year 10 students, indicating again that knowledge increased with age. Students indicated that there was consistent condom usage when they engaged in sexual intercourse, possibly implying some positive impact of good HIV and AIDS knowledge on preventive sexual behaviour.

In Guyana, the Ministry of Health, through its National AIDS Programme Secretariat (2008), conducted a cross-sectional behavioural surveillance survey of 4,600 persons comprising SW, MSM, in-school young people, out-of-school young people and the uniformed services to assess changes in their HIV and AIDS related attitudes and risk behaviours. While this survey covered diverse groups, this paper's focus was only on the in-school and out-of-school young people, since its study participants were high school students. The findings showed that 18% of out-of-school young people used marijuana; 21% of out-of-school and 25% of in-school young people indicated that they experienced forced sex; in excess of 50% of out-of-school young people said that they used condoms when engaging with transactional and regular partners; 39% of in-school young people indicated that they always used condoms with transactional partners and 49% did so with regular partners. Seventy-five per cent of out-of-school and 52% of in-school young people had HIV and AIDS knowledge on prevention pertaining to abstinence, condom usage, and being with one uninfected faithful sexual partner. Sixty-one per cent out-of-school and 71% in-school young people knew that a person can be asymptomatic with HIV infection and showed no misconception that HIV transmission can happen through mosquitoes or sharing a meal with an HIV-positive person.

Religious groups can also have an impact on HIV and AIDS knowledge. WhileZuckerman (2000) noted that African American faith-based organizations are the mainstay of the African community, another study (Griffith et al. 2010) lamented their incapacity to address the prevention needs of the HIV crisis. The most important barrier against African American faith-based organizations affecting a powerful answer to HIV is the harmful moral and religious attitudes and behaviours relating to HIV transmission (Francis andLiverpool 2009). There is a view that the relationship between religious affiliation, education, HIV and AIDS knowledge, and HIV-related sexual behaviours among African church youth was inadequately recognized (Noden et al. 2009). They conducted a study among 522 young people aged 12 to 28 in rural central Mozambique and found that religious affiliation, possibly through education delivered from the religious-affiliated schools, contributed to an increase in HIV transmission-and-prevention knowledge, but failed to impact HIV-related sexual behaviours.

In Flint, Michigan, Your Blessed Health (YBH) was a six-month pilot study to enhance the capacity of faith-based institutions and faith leaders to address HIV, AIDS and sexually transmitted infections (STIs) afflicting African American adolescents aged 11 to 19 (Griffith et al. 2010). Griffith et al. (2010, 10) noted that the YBH HIV-prevention efforts were viable and well received, provided they complied with these principles: "(1) respect the denominational doctrines and visions of the pastors, (2) engage pastors' spouses (or some other group as champions), and (3) build on the church leadership teams' understanding of what is appropriate and will be acceptable in their specific organizations".Francis et al. (2009) examined African American faith-based leaders' beliefs and attitudes in offering HIV prevention education and services to adolescents. They found that leaders expressed a keenness to deliver abstinence messages and that they would address concerns pertaining to health education but would not respond well to issues relating to HIV and AIDS.

A Trinidad & Tobago study (Genrich and Braithwaite 2005) that examined a similar type of uneasiness toward addressing HIV and AIDS complexity, defined the Hindu representative's position as: "The Hindu representative felt that HIV/AIDS occurred primarily among homosexuals and did not pose a significant problem for the Hindu organization." Furthermore, it was assumed that Hindus were less likely to acquire HIV due to high social and spiritual obligations to obey religious doctrine. According to the interviewee, HIV and AIDS was a medical problem. Although prayers and mantras are effective treatments and cures for disease, the organization was less concerned about bodily ailments than it is about eternal life. The interviewee felt that individuals living with HIV or AIDS in the Hindu community may feel discriminated against and ostracized because disease is considered an "unhygienic situation". Individuals living with HIV or AIDS are considered unclean and would be expected to stay away from organized worship. Compassion is inherent in Hinduism, but the religious groups do not provide the opportunity for confession and reconciliation.

This Trinidad & Tobago study noted uneasiness to address HIV and AIDS complexities not only from the Hindu representative, but also from some Christian denominations, such as the Open Bible, Unity of Women and Seventh Day Adventist, and from a sect within Islam, the Jamaat al Muslimeen. In contrast, adolescents in Jamaica who were committed to the church had good knowledge of HIV and AIDS (Robillard 2001).

Francis andLiverpool (2009) noted that in the US, HIV infection disproportionately impacts people of colour. HIV rates in the US have risen among adolescents, even though 89% of the schools provide educational programmes, and while African American adolescents constitute 15% of the adolescent population, they represent 61% of the AIDS rates among adolescents. African American adolescents (aged 13–18) also had limited HIV and AIDS knowledge, as girls and boys had 55% and 50% of correct scores, respectively, and showed the least knowledge on condom use and HIV testing in a study conducted by Swenson et al. (2009). A study by Glenn andWilson (2008) explored barriers to prevention interventions that may have links with a failure to design educational programmes founded on cultural competencies of the key populations vulnerable to HIV; these may relate to the cultural competencies of the key populations, such as adolescents. They recommended that information on high risk behaviour and resilience factors relating to a cultural perspective can be applied to design effective curricula and interventions to prevent HIV.

Framing appropriate curricula may improve knowledge of HIV and AIDS. A study (Holtzman et al. 1994) was administered using national probability samples of US high school students in 1989 (n = 8,098) and 1990 (n = 11,631) from grades 9 through 12 to determine changes in knowledge of HIV and AIDS, among other things. The findings showed that those students with greater knowledge of HIV and AIDS in both 1989 and 1990 were less likely to have multiple sexual partners and to engage in intravenous drug use. Additionally, school-based education and knowledge of HIV and AIDS reduced risk behaviours.

Al-Iryani et al. (2009) administered a cross-sectional study on students' knowledge of HIV and AIDS and students' stigmatizing attitudes toward PLHIV. The sample population comprised 2,274 male and female students, randomly selected from twenty-seven high schools in Aden, Yemen. The findings showed limited HIV and AIDS knowledge in prevention, such as use of condoms, with high levels of misconceptions and myths about modes of HIV transmission.

A cross-sectional study (McManus and Dhar 2008) was conducted among 251 female students from two senior secondary schools in South Delhi, India, to determine their knowledge, perceptions and attitudes toward STIs and HIV; safer sex practice and sex education; and their present sexual behaviours. One-third of these students had no sense of the signs and symptoms of STIs, except for HIV; about a third believed that HIV was curable; almost half thought that condoms should not be made available to young people; again, almost half of these students expressed confusion as to whether contraceptive pills could guard against HIV infection; and a third believed that only married women should take such pills. This study demonstrated the great need for gender-based education on STIs and HIV.

Pramanik et al. (2006) researched HIV and AIDS stigma-related attitudes among middle-class high school students in New Delhi. This cross-sectional study of 186 students found that students had limited knowledge about HIV and AIDS. Nonetheless, those with greater exposure to HIV and AIDS education had greater knowledge than those without the exposure. Males with more exposure to HIV and AIDS education had better knowledge of HIV and AIDS than females.

A study in San Francisco (DiClemente et al. 1986) found that most of the students, both males and females, knew that sexual intercourse was one of the modes of HIV transmission, but only about two-thirds knew that using a condom during sexual intercourse would reduce the risk of contracting HIV infection. They suggested that a teaching module on HIV education be included in the school curriculum. In another study, DiClemente et al. (1988) found that more white than black and Latino adolescents in San Francisco high schools knew that using condoms during sexual intercourse would reduce the risk of HIV transmission. Blacks were almost twice as likely to harbour misconceptions about HIV and AIDS as whites, and Latinos were more than twice as likely to harbour misconceptions about HIV and AIDS as whites. Misconceptions abounded within the black group, but more so within the Latino group. In 1990, circa the time of the study, the estimated adult (15–49) HIV prevalence for the US was 0.5% (UNAIDS/WHO 2008). These San Francisco minority adolescents' understanding of the barrier method (condoms) was in tandem with their belief in the misconceptions. As of 1988, DiClemente et al.'s 1986 suggestion for incorporating HIV education in the school curriculum had not gained support.

In 2003, Savaser reported the findings of a study on 705 high school students (360 ninth graders and 345 eleventh graders; 305 females, 400 males) in Turkey to determine their knowledge of and attitudes toward HIV and AIDS. Males had higher scores than females, and eleventh graders did better than ninth graders; gender and age impacted the assimilation of HIV and AIDS knowledge. Of those surveyed, 40.3% recognized that a symptom-free carrier of HIV infection could transmit the infection; 68.5% had a strong proclivity to taking the HIV test; over half indicated that if diagnosed with HIV, they would seek hospital assistance; and about half did not recognize that young people and hospital workers could be part of a risk group. Savaser found that private school students had higher knowledge of HIV and AIDS than public school students. There seemed to be a better understanding of the modes of transmission than modes of non-transmission. Turkey remains a low prevalence country in Central

Europe, with an HIV adult (15–49) prevalence of <0.1% in 2009 (UNAIDS Narrative Report-Turkey 2010).

A study (Macchi et al. 2008) in Asuncion and Lambare, Paraguay, found that secondary school students in the first, second and third years showed poor knowledge of HIV and AIDS. About half of these students had sexual relations, with their first sexual intercourse at an average age of 14.6, with almost three-quarters of them indicating that they knew how to conduct themselves in risk situations. In contrast, secondary school students in the Ivory Coast did not conduct themselves appropriately in risk situations; many students knew that condom use is a preventive measure, but still did not at all times use condoms, notwithstanding having good knowledge of HIV and AIDS (Toure 2005).

In Lagos, Nigeria, a study (Borire et al. 2008), using self-administered questionnaires and multistage sampling, showed statistical significance between condom usage and type of school, with the public more than the missionary school inclined to using condoms; also, there was a statistically significant relationship between type of school and number of sexual partners, again with the public school outmatching the missionary school on this front. Nevertheless, the public and missionary secondary schools showed no differences in HIV and AIDS knowledge and most students had good HIV and AIDS knowledge, crediting the mass media and their school for this information.

In Benin City, Nigeria, Wagbatsoma and Okojie (2006) did a cross-sectional study of a random sample of 852 students drawn from three secondary schools (one all-male, one all-female and one mixed) to assess their knowledge of HIV and AIDS. Many students had good awareness of HIV, but few knew its causes. About two-thirds indicated that sexual intercourse was the main transmission route, but that having multiple sexual partners was popular among the 13–15 age groups. Their poor knowledge of HIV and AIDS led them to embrace myths and misconceptions of contracting HIV, such as through kissing, living with PLHIV and sharing eating utensils of PLHIV.

There were also other situations where students had good knowledge of HIV and AIDS, yet embraced misconceptions. Caribbean African American female adolescents in South Florida, US, possessed good knowledge of HIV, but would not share space or personal belongings with PLHIV (Archibald 2007). African American adolescents in a children's homeless emergency shelter had good knowledge of HIV; nevertheless, their attitude and behaviour toward condom use bore little relationship to this knowledge (Liverpool et al. 2002).

Amoakoh-Coleman (2006) examined the HIV and STIs knowledge, attitudes and practices of 150 adolescents from five schools in Greater Accra, Ghana, using convenience sampling. She found a huge gap in knowledge, attitude and practice pertaining to HIV and STIs and that the adolescents were sexually active at an early age. There was little behavioural change as a result of the misconceptions about HIV, AIDS and STIs.

In 1999, most of the senior secondary school students in Udupi District, Karnataka, India (Agrawal et al. 1999), showed that they possessed adequate knowledge of HIV, but also harboured several misconceptions on modes of HIV transmission. Around the time of the study, the estimated adult (15–49) HIV prevalence for India was about 0.5% (UNAIDS/WHO 2008).

As in so many studies, students showed a better understanding of HIV transmission than non-transmission modes. Male secondary school students in Alkhobar, Saudi Arabia, showed good knowledge of HIV transmission modes, but the majority had poor general knowledge of HIV and AIDS (Al-Almaie 2005). A high HIV and AIDS knowledge score was significantly and positively related to class grade, Saudi nationality and high secondary level.

National-based household survey data from a cross-sectional study (Bankole et al. 2007) on adolescents aged 12 to 19 in Burkina Faso, Ghana, Malawi and Uganda found that many were already sexually active. These adolescents displayed high awareness, but had minimal in-depth knowledge about pregnancy and HIV prevention. This means that school-based sex education becomes critical for the under-15 age group.

Mushi, Mpembeni and Jahn (2007) administered a qualitative and quantitative study of 135 randomly selected students aged 9 to 17 from three primary schools in rural Tanzania to evaluate their knowledge of safe motherhood and HIV. Focus group interviews were held with thirty-five students. Students had low knowledge of safe motherhood and HIV and did not know the likely age of conception. Most believed that it was safe for a girl to become married prior to age 18, that difficulties encountered during pregnancy and delivery happened because there was no adherence to traditions and taboos. The study also found that there was little knowledge about prenatal and postpartum care and vertical HIV transmission and prevention. Again, there is great need for school-based education on safe motherhood.

A recent Iranian survey (Movahed and Shoaa 2010) examined attitudes toward HIV and AIDS and sociocultural factors of a sample of 600 high school students in Shiraz, Iran. The study presented attitudes as relating to knowledge, emotion and tendency to action. The results confirmed that about half of these students had poor knowledge of HIV and AIDS, and only about a third had moderate knowledge of HIV and AIDS. Influences on students' knowledge included study major, parent education, father's occupation, utilization of books and the internet.

Another study (Yazdi et al. 2006) was conducted among the three grades of high school students in Hashtgerd, Iran. This city had a population of 28,000 in 2002, and out of a total of eighty-one high schools, nineteen were selected with a sample of 1,227 students for the study that commenced in the same year. The study found that about 62% of adolescents possessed moderate knowledge of HIV and AIDS; females showed higher knowledge than males, but the difference was minimal. With respect to HIV transmission, over 90% of the students indicated that the most genuine modes of HIV transmission were sharing needles and razors, mother-to-child transmission, and heterosexual sex; they apportioned homosexuality with less credence for HIV transmission.

While there was moderate understanding of HIV and AIDS, there were pervasive misconceptions. For instance, about 15–30% believed that HIV infection could be contracted through casual physical contact, like hugging (27%), kissing (14%) and shaking hands, or even being in close proximity to PLHIV. Some students indicated that HIV is curable (43%) or preventable (81%) through vaccinations and avoiding people who visited PLHIV (52%). A small number believed that casual contact could transmit HIV, and about half (47%) did not endorse condom use as an effective prevention method. Significant numbers of students indicated that sharing a toothbrush, sharing scissors, drinking from the same glass, using public toilets, sharing razors, sharing tattoo instruments and sharing dentistry instruments could lead to HIV infection. Some misconceptions about the modes of HIV transmission were similar to the findings in Tavoosi et al.'s study (2004), such as mosquito bites (33%), public swimming pools (21%) and public restrooms (20%). Yazdi et al. (2006) recommended prevention education in schools, and reviewed how cultural and religious values bear upon people's lifestyles and information access.

A study among secondary school students in Ogun State, Nigeria (Odusanya and Bankole 2006) reported the findings on students' knowledge and awareness of sexually transmitted infections, and the general beliefs and attitudes associated with HIV infection and PLHIV. Of those surveyed, 85.2% recognized that gonorrhoea is an STI; 62.9% recognized that syphilis is an STI; 22.2% felt that they had much knowledge of HIV and AIDS; 63.0% indicated that they possessed moderate knowledge of HIV and AIDS; 77.8% correctly recognized HIV as a viral infection; 85.5% recognized that HIV is incurable; 75% were aware that there is no vaccine for HIV; 90% knew that PLHIV typically appeared healthy; 85.7% recognized having multiple sexual partners as a means of HIV transmission; 90% knew that a person could contract HIV from infected blood and other infected blood products; and 77.3% and 72.4% brought up unsterilized needles and dental equipment, respectively, as likely sources of HIV transmission. With regard to prevention modes against contracting HIV, 88.9% referred to abstinence from sex, 83.8% mentioned condom use and 74.3% talked about not having sex with commercial workers. In 2006, circa the time of the study, the estimated adult (15–49) HIV prevalence for Nigeria was 3% (UNAIDS/WHO 2008). The study found several deficiencies in awareness, and suggested the need to embed awareness programmes in the school curriculum.

Throughout the literature, adolescents generally showed a basic knowledge of the modes of HIV transmission. In 2007, Manji et al. (2007) reported that over 90% of adolescents in a study among Nicaragua's male and female adolescents understood that vaginal sex is a mode of HIV transmission. However, only a little over half recognized that anal sex and oral sex are also modes of HIV infection, and that apparently healthy, but HIV-infected, persons can also transmit the virus. Just over 75% had correct knowledge about the myths of HIV transmission. There were no differences in HIV knowledge among both male and female adolescents.

In 2007, circa the time of the study, the estimated adult (15–49) HIV prevalence for Nicaragua was 0.2% (UNAIDS/WHO 2008). The fact that Nicaraguan adolescents had good general and prevention HIV knowledge might indicate the potency of sex education programmes in positively impacting HIV transmission, notwithstanding their limitations in Nicaragua. Nonetheless, the fact that education did not produce the desired effect in reducing HIV infection in other countries might indicate the need to identify any distinctive form and content of Nicaragua's sex education programmes which may hold a promise for those countries.

Rondini and Krugu (2009) conducted a study on secondary school students in the Bolgatanga community in Northern Ghana to ascertain their knowledge, attitudes and reproductive health practices. These students had limited knowledge concerning family planning methods and modes of HIV transmission, and the fact that they showed little inclination to use contraceptives placed them at high risk for unwanted pregnancies and HIV infection. Clearly, limited accessibility and poor infrastructure placed rural Northern Ghana at high risk for HIV infection.

Kozlova, Nizharadze and Polyakova (2004) administered a study comprising semi-structured interviews and evaluating structured inventories to ascertain sexual behaviours, injecting drug use, knowledge and representations of HIV transmission among school and shelter youth in Russia, Georgia and Ukraine. Shelter youth were more likely than school youth to engage in injecting drug use and to have sex; Georgian school youth more than the other school youth were likely to have sex and participate in injecting drug use; and shelter youth and Georgians were more likely than the others to have misconceptions about HIV. School-based HIV interventions are critical for the Russian and Ukrainian shelter youth and Georgian school youth. Both the out-of-school young people in the Guyana Ministry of Health study (2008) and shelter youth in Russia, Georgia and Ukraine displayed similar drug-taking behaviours; the shelter youth in Russia, Georgia and Ukraine, and about a third of out-of-school and a quarter of in-school youth in the Guyana Ministry of Health sample expressed similar misconceptions about HIV and AIDS.

In 2005, in another part of the globe, South Korean high school students (Yoo et al. 2005) showed only a moderate knowledge of HIV and AIDS with average scores of 13.93 out of 19 for male students and 13.35 for female students. For those who engaged in sexual intercourse, less than half of these used condoms. This finding is not surprising because about half of the students showed reticent concern for HIV, as more than half of these students believed that casual contact is a mode of HIV transmission. In 2005, the estimated adult (15–49 age group) HIV prevalence for South Korea was about 0.1% (World Bank 2011). The finding of a low prevalence and infrequent use of condoms in South Korea might signify that adolescents had stable sex partners.

In 1994, a study showed that a huge number of Kenyan high school students (77.1%) with adequate knowledge of HIV engaged in extensive sexual experience without using condoms (Pattullo et al. 1994). Nevertheless, Kenyan students showed knowledge of HIV as demonstrated by the following: the incapacity of mosquitoes to transmit HIV, failure of condoms to protect, failure of medications to protect, the terminal and incurable aspect of AIDS, and the healthy appearance of those with HIV. In 1994, the estimated adult (15–49) HIV prevalence for Kenya was unavailable, but when it became available in 2001, it was around 8% (UNAIDS/WHO 2008). The reported behaviours of the Kenyan students showed similarities with African American and Latino students, Iranian students, and Portuguese students, particularly with regard to myths and misconceptions of HIV transmission.

Misconceptions, however, were endemic in Iran. A cluster sampling study on grade two high school students in Tehran, Iran (Tavoosi et al. 2004) found that while most of the students from a sample of 4,641 from 52 out of a total of 500 secondary schools had good knowledge of HIV, they still embraced the following misconceptions: children were not likely to contract HIV; PLHIV can be recognized by their appearance; there was a cure for AIDS and the AIDS vaccine was available; and HIV infection could emanate from hugging, kissing, using public toilets, using public swimming pools, coughing and sneezing, dentistry, and mosquito bites. In 2004, circa the time of the study, the estimated adult (15–49) HIV prevalence for Iran was about 0.2% (UNAIDS/WHO 2008). Perhaps, we could assume that in Iran, misconceptions contributed to reduced HIV transmission. The Islamic religious beliefs and an intolerant attitude toward PLHIV, too, may explain the low prevalence in Iran.

In a US study, there were significant differences in the mean knowledge scores among seniors from different ethnic groups (Hancock et al. 1999). African American seniors had the lowest mean knowledge score while White seniors had the highest mean knowledge score. Both freshman and senior students had misconceptions on modes of transmission, prevention methods for sexual transmission of HIV, the significance of HIV antibody testing, the transmission of HIV through body fluids and the common causes of death for those afflicted with AIDS. In 1999, circa the time of the study, the estimated adult (15–49) HIV prevalence for the U.S. was 0.6% (UNAIDS/WHO 2008).

DiClemente et al. (1987) conducted an early study to review HIV and AIDS knowledge, beliefs and attitudes among adolescents, and found that a large number of adolescents expressed fears about contracting HIV. They suggested that HIV risk-reduction programmes would require dispelling myths and misconceptions about HIV infection, and particularly those myths pertaining to casual contagion of the infection. They also argued that adolescents carrying such misconceptions may embrace fear and anxiety about personal susceptibility to contracting HIV, and removing misconceptions may decrease such fear and anxiety vis-à-vis stigmatizing PLHIV.

A sample of Portuguese from the WHO collaborative research (Currie et al. 2001) "Health Behaviour in School-Aged Children 2002 (HBSC)" (Matos and Aventura 2003) provided the basis for a study of Portuguese adolescents (Dias et al. 2006). These adolescents were aware that using contaminated needles and engaging in sexual intercourse with an HIV-infected woman are modes of HIV transmission; just under half of them did not believe that coughing and sneezing could produce HIV infection, and about half believed that oral contraceptives could not serve as a barrier against HIV infection. More females than males showed greater knowledge of HIV, and the higher age group (10th grade) had good knowledge as well.

Yet, undefined fears characterized this group, and despite good knowledge of the modes of HIV transmission, many of them still had concerns about the potency of the myths and misconceptions about HIV transmission. In 2006, circa the time of the study, the estimated adult (15–49) HIV prevalence for Portugal was 0.5% (UNAIDS/WHO 2008). In Portugal, each student has a right to sex education through the 3/84 Law of 1984 and the 120/99 Law of 1999 that stipulated the presentation of general topics (Nodin et al. 2004); but sex education was not standardized, and its presentation in the classroom was left to teachers and other organizations' initiatives. Clearly, the fact that good HIV knowledge among Portuguese adolescents failed to eliminate their concerns about misconceptions seemed to raise questions about the quality of education as a preventative measure.

Most students had knowledge of the disease in a study of HIV knowledge, beliefs, attitudes and practices of adolescents in two senior secondary schools in Jamnagar, Gujarat, India (Bhalla et al. 2005). There were no differences between the biology and non-biology stream students: both groups of students embraced myths and misconceptions of HIV.

The Division of Adolescent and School Health of the Centers for Disease Control and Prevention conducted a national study of the data from the Secondary School Student Health Risk Survey (SSSHRS) (Anderson et al. 1990). They found that most of the high school students who had prior HIV education in school in comparison with those who had none were more familiar with the two main modes of HIV transmission – intravenous drug use and sexual intercourse. Those with prior HIV education also reported not having more than two sexual partners and consistently used condoms. Females had higher HIV knowledge scores than males. Other literature shows that Indian students, African American and Latino students, Portuguese students, and Iranian students had moderate to good knowledge of HIV transmission, but harboured myths and misconceptions of HIV transmission. Perhaps students with good knowledge of HIV who harboured myths and misconceptions might not have had the benefit of prior HIV education in school.

Mahat and Scoloveno (2006) reported their findings on HIV knowledge, attitudes and beliefs of adolescents in Nepal. The study showed that the participants had a moderate general knowledge of HIV and that males had greater knowledge of HIV than females. However, their study revealed that participants had knowledge deficiencies with respect to modes of HIV transmission and prevention. In 2006, circa the time of the study, the estimated adult (15–49) HIV prevalence for Nepal was 0.5% (UNAIDS/WHO 2008). They found that most Nepalese adolescents who thought that HIV was a huge problem were afraid of contracting the infection, and most indicated that they would take an HIV test if it were without cost. Some felt, too, that they would not contract the infection.

Another study assessed and compared knowledge of HIV between high-school freshmen and senior-level students to determine the correlation between demographics and students' knowledge level (Hancock et al. 1999). These students were from one county in Central California. There was no significant difference in knowledge level between male and female freshman students, but there was a significant difference between the genders among senior students' knowledge level. Female more than male seniors had higher knowledge level scores on HIV.

Goodman and Cohall (1989) conducted a study on HIV among inner city adolescents (n = 196) in New York City. There was good knowledge of HIV modes of transmission, and sexual behaviours were found to be the most significant risk factor for HIV: 58% engaged in sexual intercourse, with 12% using no contraceptive method, and no injecting drug use was reported.

Many studies in this section show that good knowledge of HIV and AIDS does not necessarily lead to behaviour change of adolescents' negative attitudes toward PLHIV. For this reason, the next focus is to review studies on stigma-related attitudes, as stigma has become a significant barrier against reducing HIV transmission.

Stigma-related Attitudes/Perceptions

Sallar (2009) found that in Ghana there were statistically significant associations between misconceptions and myths, and negative attitudes toward PLHIV. Out-of-school adolescents had less caring attitudes toward relatives with HIV or AIDS, would let PLHIV hide their status, would let them have employment, were not keen on PLHIV to have appropriate health care and said that PLHIV should be secluded. Clearly, out-of-school adolescents were strong catalysts for reinforcing stigma. The Ministry of Health through the National AIDS Programme Secretariat (2008) in Guyana found high levels of HIV and AIDS-related stigmatized attitudes among out-of-school and in-school young people. The Al-Iryani et al. study (2009) also found that the students driving up high levels of stigma and discrimination in Aden, Yemen, were those with limited knowledge of HIV.

A questionnaire study (El-Gadi S. et al. 2008) among high school students in the North West of Libya found both male and female students to be projecting high stigmatized behaviours; nonetheless, most of the students also supported the provision of free care to PLHIV. Culture also became a barrier for reducing stigma toward PLHIV; some studies indicated that the more the Native American related to his/her culture, the more there was negativity in attitudes toward HIV, AIDS and Hepatitis C virus (HCV) (Bertolli et al. 2004). Earlier in this chapter, studies of different religious sects were presented showing some ambivalence toward HIV, AIDS and PLHIV, a finding quite consistent with this Native American study.

Manji, Pena and Dubrow (2007) found that adolescents in Leon, Nicaragua had positive attitudes toward PLHIV. About 90% of them would care for a family member with HIV or AIDS, about 71% would provide care for a friend and just under half of them would share food with PLHIV. In addition, adolescents in Nicaragua saw condom usage as reducing sexual pleasure; displayed machismo attitudes toward gender roles in sex; assumed that a woman should have sexual relations only if married, or if she has a stable partner; assumed that an unmarried man has nothing to lose if he has sex and is not in a relationship; assumed that a woman can negotiate with a man to use a condom during sex; assumed that a man can use a condom during sex without it being seen as mistrust from his partner; and held that women and men can, without restraint, experience and enjoy sex.

A Nigerian study (Odusanya and Bankole 2006) showed that 48.8% of students would have no proclivity to eat off a clean plate or drink from the same cup that an HIV-infected person used, 41.1% believed that HIV-infected students should not attend school, 40.2% felt that PLHIV should not remain at work and 35.5% indicated that they would end their relationship with an HIV-infected friend.

Students in Tehran high schools expressed negative attitudes toward PLHIV (Tavoosi et al. 2004). Both males and females believed that HIV-infected persons should not attend school, and 23% of students would not shake hands with an HIV-infected person if they knew upfront that the individual was HIV-positive. There was a correlation between attitude and knowledge in that the lower the knowledge of HIV, the greater the negative attitude. Also, about half the students would show compassion for PLHIV, and females would tend to express greater compassion than males toward PLHIV. Another Iranian study (Movahed and Shoaa 2010) indicated that only 15.4% of Iranian students in Shiraz City had positive attitudes toward HIV and AIDS. They found that affinity to Islamic religious beliefs, major of study, gender, mother's occupation and some mass media significantly impacted students' attitudes toward HIV and AIDS.

In the Turkey study (Savaser 2003), half of the high school students believed PLHIV should attend school, and that they should not cease working. Adolescents in Jamaica tended to show less sympathy toward PLHIV, condemned sexual relations between two men and sexual relations between two women, and harboured fear and negative feelings toward PLHIV (Norman, Carr and Jiménez 2006).

In the South Korean study (Yoo et al. 2005), female students showed fewer proclivities than males to care for any significant others with AIDS, were less willing to care for those with HIV even occasionally and endorsed the residential quarantine of persons with HIV or AIDS. In Agrawal et al.'s cross-sectional study (1999) of 990 students and 46 trainee teachers in Karnataka, India, health talks and a hand-out made a positive difference in students' attitudes to HIV. Saudi Arabian secondary school students showed inappropriate attitudes toward HIV and AIDS, and only high secondary level students showed a positive and significant relationship with appropriate attitudes toward HIV and AIDS (Al-Almaie 2005).

Dias et al.'s study (2006) of Portuguese adolescents found that despite their understanding that a lack of knowledge would make people feel uncomfortable toward people living with HIV, they still harboured undefined fears of the disease. These were ambivalent attitudes that made people feel uncomfortable among PLHIV, and some of them would ostracize PLHIV and would not share the same room with that person. These adolescents with ambivalent attitudes possibly had deficiencies in their knowledge of modes of HIV transmission. Dias et al. (2006) noted that those who had good knowledge of modes of HIV transmission would tend to evolve positive attitudes toward PLHIV. Female adolescents had greater knowledge of modes of HIV transmission and tended to present positive attitudes toward PLHIV. Adolescents in Portugal surmised that AIDS is dangerous, lethal and incurable; perceived PLHIV as suffering from discrimination and social exclusion; recognized that limited knowledge contributed to discrimination against PLHIV; and expressed greater sympathy toward PLHIV. Overall, adolescents had positive attitudes toward PLHIV. On the contrary, in Swaziland coeducational secondary schools, students with good knowledge of HIV and AIDS and increased peer influence had reduced stigmatizing attitudes (Buseh et al. 2006), but those students who felt susceptible tended to show greater HIV and AIDS stigma-related attitudes.

Yazdi et al. (2006) found that 90% of the students in Hashtgerd, Iran, saw HIV and AIDS as a huge problem. They appreciated media activities to raise awareness and believed that discussing HIV and AIDS would hardly be expected to increase its prevalence. Most Iranian students had negative attitudes toward PLHIV. These students agreed that HIV testing should become mandatory before marriage. About half of them felt that HIV-positive people should face quarantine, one-third believed that HIV is a sin and just under half believed that HIV is curable. In 2006, circa the time of this study, the estimated adult (15–49) HIV prevalence for Iran was about 0.2% (UNAIDS/WHO 2008). One can reason, then, that in Iran, moderate knowledge of HIV and AIDS and a low prevalence might suggest that education had minimum effect on HIV transmission, and that perhaps the influencing factor in explaining the low prevalence might be students' Islamic religious beliefs that guided their thinking on HIV and on premarital sex.

A Kenyan study (Pattullo et al. 1994) found that about 20% of Kenyan high school students believed that PLHIV should not be provided with employment; about a third believed that they should be quarantined; two-thirds believed that PLHIV were to be blamed for contracting the infection; and 88.2% believed that PLHIV should be treated with compassion, quite contradictory to the other attitudes pertaining to employment, quarantine and blaming PLHIV. This study suggested that students' contradictory attitudes might be related to their concerns about casual contact and the possibility of contracting the infection.

Interventions to Increase Knowledge of HIV and AIDS

Children of migrant Chinese workers enhanced their knowledge of HIV and AIDS, changed their attitude and boosted their protection self-efficacy after receiving three months of peer-education-based HIV and AIDS intervention using the interactive method (Li et al. 2010). Li et al. conducted a study of peer-led intervention on children of migrant workers in China and found that after three months of intervention, the adolescents knew how to prevent HIV infection, were more likely to care for PLHIV, alleviated their fear of AIDS and developed awareness in an HIV and AIDS-friendly environment.

In Fujian Province, China, a peer-led HIV prevention education as an intervention among senior high school students increased their knowledge of reproductive health, HIV and AIDS, and sexually transmitted infections (Ye et al. 2009). This was a two-year follow-up study from March 2006 through April 2008, and comprised 3,068 students from fourteen schools in 2006, and 893 students from five schools represented the follow-up group. This study was one of the few in China that examined the long-term consequences of a prevention intervention programme among Chinese high school students.

Cai et al.'s study (2008) among 1,950 students from ten senior high schools in Shanghai, China, also found that peer-education-based HIV and AIDS intervention increased knowledge of HIV and AIDS as well as modified long-term behavioural intention. Shen et al. (2008) also reviewed peer education methods in HIV prevention intervention among ten different senior high schools in Shanghai. These were three key, four ordinary, and three vocational senior high schools. It was found that the peer education method was useful, but that each type of school should have different content and schedules and that the vocational school would need greater inputs of health education.

Huang et al. (2008) examined the usefulness of peer-led prevention intervention on HIV and AIDS knowledge, attitudes and behavioural intention among senior high school students in San-Ming, China. A total of 3,068 students completed a self-administered questionnaire for pre- and post-intervention, and 981 students constituted the intervention group exposed to the peer-led intervention, while the rest of the students comprised the control group that followed the regular teacher-led health education programme. They found that the peer-led intervention was valuable in terms of improving HIV and AIDS knowledge, attitudes and behavioural intention for the intervention group. There were some variations in HIV and AIDS knowledge and attitudes pertaining to gender, health education history and pedagogical methods.

Cheng et al. (2008) conducted a quasi-experimental study among rural senior high school students in Shangcai County, China, to determine the usefulness of an intervention with a life-planning skills programme and participatory training methods. After three months, the life-skills training programme improved HIV and AIDS knowledge, attitudes, protection self-efficacy and communication among these senior high school students. A study (Abdullah et al. 2003) conducted in Hong Kong also found that an educational talk as an intervention resulted in an increase in Chinese high school students' knowledge of HIV and AIDS.

Al-Iryani et al. (2011) administered a study that evaluated the effectiveness of a school-based peer education programme to improve HIV knowledge on transmission modes and prevention in twenty-seven secondary schools in Aden, Yemen. The peer education intervention programme resulted in 62.8% of the students developing a good HIV knowledge score on transmission modes and prevention, and 71.2% of females had better knowledge scores than their male counterparts with 54.7%. The peer education programme also reduced misconceptions.

Barss et al. (2009) conducted a peer-based education intervention study among 1,398 female and 505 male high school students from two major cities of the United Arab Emirates. The 90-minute intervention comprised factual information and three attitude workshops. Females showed more or less reduced baseline HIV knowledge than males, but showed increased improvement with the intervention in both knowledge and attitude.

The Lagos State Ministry of Education in Nigeria introduced Family Life and HIV Education Curriculum to government junior secondary school students in 2003 (Esiet et al. 2009). In November 2004, the knowledge and attitudes of 1,366 students were measured at the start of the school year, and again at the end of the school year in July 2005. The curriculum intervention worked, as those exposed to the curriculum improved their knowledge of sexuality and HIV, and provided support for abstinence and gender equality.

Ngao was an HIV education intervention programme administered in the mid-1990s in Tanzania to cultivate positive attitudes of 814 students in grades 6 and 7 toward PLHIV, and to reduce intentions to be sexually active in the near-term. A controlled group randomized trial (Stigler et al. 2006) was used to evaluate the efficacy of this intervention twelve months after the baseline. The results indicated that that increased exposure to HIV and AIDS information and increased knowledge about HIV transmission/ prevention were significant mediators of the intervention's impact to reduce the stigmatized effect on PLHIV. A case was made here for school-based HIV education interventions.

In a Hong Kong study (Lau, Tsui and Chan 2005), intervention effects were stronger among female students than among male students. Prior to the intervention, 17.3% of participants showed no proclivity to initiate personal contacts with PLHIV, but this percentage declined to 6.4% after the intervention. Also, prior to the intervention, some 40% advocated for a law to prohibit PLHIV from engaging in sexual activities, but after the intervention this fell to 20%.

Relationship between HIV and AIDS Knowledge and Stigma-related Attitudes/Perceptions

Limited HIV and AIDS knowledge resulting in risk behaviours and stigmatization of PLHIV has posed formidable difficulties for young people to protect themselves from the disease (Aggarwal Sharma and Chhabra 2000; Sullivan et al. 2010; Wu et al. 2007). Although the relationship between HIV knowledge and attitude and behaviour change is not definitive, the Western world still views HIV knowledge as a significant variable for effective prevention (Ajzen 1991; Fisher and Fisher 1992).

This study also shares the view on the significance of HIV knowledge for prevention intervention effectiveness. It also shows that the sample of high school students only have moderate HIV and AIDS knowledge, contradicting a previous study's finding (GDHS 2009) that people's knowledge of HIV and AIDS in Guyana is high. In fact, the GDHS study only used two dimensions of HIV and AIDS knowledge: whether people have heard about HIV and AIDS, and their knowledge of two prevention methods – condom use and limiting sexual intercourse to one faithful uninfected partner. This study used seven dimensions of HIV and AIDS knowledge. However, there has been no comprehensive study on the level of HIV and AIDS knowledge and the relationship between this knowledge and stigma-related attitudes in Guyana.

A cross-sectional study (Qu et al. 2010) examined the association between 528 student nurses' HIV and AIDS knowledge and attitudes by applying a structural equation model (SEM). These students were at the technical secondary school of the China Medical University. The findings showed that specialty knowledge, negative attitude, knowledge of transmission routes and knowledge of non-transmission routes impacted directly and indirectly on occupational attitude. The study also found that preventive knowledge and positive attitude minimally impacted occupational attitude. These findings suggested that student nurses should change their occupational attitude through gaining specialty knowledge, knowledge of transmission and non-transmission routes, and minimize their negative attitudes toward HIV and AIDS.

Another cross-sectional study (Bhowon and Ah-Kion 2005) examined the knowledge and attitudes of 160 youth in Mauritius. The study found that about half of the youth showed moderate knowledge of HIV and

AIDS, and about half had liberal attitudes toward PLHIV. However, there was no significant relationship between knowledge and attitudes, suggesting that having knowledge of HIV and AIDS did not necessarily generate liberal attitudes toward PLHIV.

Walusimbi and Okonski (2004) conducted a cross-sectional study of 557 licensed nurses and midwives in Uganda in 2001 to assess their HIV and AIDS knowledge and attitudes. The study found a correlation between high HIV and AIDS knowledge and positive attitudes, indicating that the higher the knowledge level, the greater the positive attitudes. There was a significant negative correlation between knowledge scores and fear of contagion, meaning that the higher the knowledge level, the lower the fear of contagion.

Tebourski and Alaya (2004) reported on a survey administered in the capital of Tunisia among high school students in 2002. The study showed that students had good knowledge of the modes of HIV transmission, but had a misconception on the role of condoms, mistaken views about the HIV transmission mode and negative attitudes toward PLHIV. The study also found no correlation between knowledge and attitudes toward PLHIV. Religion appeared to be the major influencing factor on students' attitudes toward PLHIV.

Nwokocha and Nwakoby (2002) conducted a cross-sectional study of 360 high school students from five secondary schools in Enugu, Nigeria to assess their knowledge, attitude and behaviour regarding HIV and AIDS. Students had a defective understanding of HIV and AIDS, and were scared of the disease because it is deadly and has no cure; they did not know about the cause, nature and transmission modes of the disease. The students' defective knowledge produced inappropriate attitudes and behaviours toward HIV and AIDS.

A cross-sectional study (Lahai-Momoh and Ross 1997) of 137 high school students aged 14 and over from two high schools in Bo and Freetown, Sierra Leone, investigated the relationship between their HIV and AIDS knowledge, attitudes and perceptions. The study found no significant differences in HIV and AIDS knowledge scores by age, factor score, sex, intercourse or condom use.

Summary of HIV and AIDS Knowledge and Stigma-related Attitudes/Perceptions

A number of studies showed adolescents with moderate to good knowledge of HIV and AIDS, with no sex differences in knowledge (Di Clemente et al. 1986, 1988; Pattullo et al. 1994; Agrawal et al. 1999; Tavoosi et al. 2004; Yoo et al. 2005; Yazdi et al. 2006; Odusanya and Bankole 2006; Manji et al. 2007; Movahed and Shoaa 2010).

Then there were other studies that showed adolescents with moderate to good knowledge of HIV and AIDS, with sex differences in knowledge (Anderson et al. 1990; Hancock et al. 1999; Al-Iryani et al. 2011; Rossem et al. 2010; Dias et al. 2006; Mahat and Scoloveno 2006; Savaser 2003). The Portugal study (Dias et al. 2006) showed that there were more females than males with good knowledge of HIV and AIDS. The Nepal study (Mahat and Scoloveno 2006) and the Turkey study (Savaser 2003) indicated that more males than females had moderate knowledge of HIV and AIDS.

There were also studies that showed that increased age led to an increase in knowledge (Dias et al. 2006; Hancock et al. 1999; Savaser 2003; Rossem, Berten and Tuyckom 2010; Agius et al. 2010).

Several studies also revealed that some students who had good knowledge of HIV and AIDS also harboured misconceptions, myths and fears about HIV and AIDS (DiClemente, Zorn and Temoshok 1986; Dias et al. 2006; DiClemente et al. 1988; Tavoosi et al. 2004; Yazdi et al. 2006; Pattullo et al. 1994; Agrawal et al. 1999; Hancock et al. 1999; Mahat and Scoloveno 2006; Norman, Carr and Jiménez 2006).

This literature review showed more negative than positive attitudes of adolescents toward HIV, AIDS and PLHIV. Studies that showed positive attitudes also showed moderate to good knowledge of HIV and AIDS among adolescents (Dias et al. 2006; Savaser 2003; Lau, Tsui and Chan 2005; Manji, Pena and Dubrow 2007; Li et al. 2010). Some of the adolescents' positive attitudes toward PLHIV included the following: that PLHIV should attend school and stay in employment, their interest in taking the HIV test, their proclivity to initiate personal contact with PLHIV, no law to prohibit PLHIV's sexual activities, care for a family member, care for a friend, sharing food with PLHIV, less fear of AIDS, and developing awareness in an HIV-friendly environment.

There were also studies that showed negative perceptions even when the study indicated moderate to good knowledge of HIV and AIDS among adolescents (Yazdi et al. 2006; Tavoosi et al. 2004; Movahed and Shoaa 2010; Yoo et al. 2005; Pattullo et al. 1994; Mahat and Scoloveno 2006; Odusanya and Bankole 2006; Norman, Carr and Jimenez 2006). Some of the adolescents' negative (and sometimes incorrect) perceptions of PLHIV included the following: AIDS is lethal and incurable, mandatory HIV testing should be conducted before marriage, PLHIV should be quarantined, HIV is a sin and curable, handshakes with PLHIV must be avoided, and PLHIV should not gain employment. The adolescents surveyed also expressed unwillingness to care for PLHIV as a significant other or as a friend; they blamed PLHIV for their plight; they viewed HIV and AIDS as a huge problem; they expressed fear of contracting HIV; they indicated their unwillingness to eat from a clean plate or drink from the same cup as PLHIV; they indicated that they would end relationships with PLHIV; and they showed little sympathy for PLHIV, particularly MSM and Women Sex Workers (WSW).

Notwithstanding the negative attitudes among some adolescents in Iran (Tavoosi et al. 2004) and Kenya (Pattullo et al. 1994), they still expressed compassion for PLHIV. Pattullo et al. (1994) argued that this contradictory emotion occurred possibly because of lingering fears of casual contact leading to HIV infection. There also were some ambivalent attitudes – uncomfortable with, ostracism for and not wanting to share a room with PLHIV – among Portuguese adolescents (Dias et al. 2006). This ambivalence may pertain to gaps in knowledge about HIV transmission modes because misconceptions could breed stigmatizing responses (Dias et al. 2006). Herek et al. (2002) also noted that understanding behaviours pertaining to HIV transmission may reduce stigmatizing attitudes toward PLHIV. Francis and Liverpool (2009) observed the severity of HIV among African Americans, especially adolescents. They advocated non-traditional intervention methods vis-à-vis faith-based organizations, which by engaging a huge cross-section of the African American community can disseminate HIV prevention strategies and messages. Church- and faith-based organizations and African Americans as people of colour have to become long-term interlocking partners in a critical struggle to end HIV infection within their communities. Other faith-based communities may also have to engage themselves in order to prevent further transmission of HIV.

The Theory of Planned Behaviour (TPB) as an Explanatory Model for Findings in the Literature Review

The TPB (Ajzen 2006) constitutes a useful model for explaining the relationship between HIV and AIDS knowledge and attitude-related stigma among high school students toward PLHIV, HIV and AIDS in the literature review.

Figure 2.1 presents three concerns that direct human behaviour – behavioural beliefs, normative beliefs and control beliefs.

A behavioural belief is the probability that a behaviour will generate a particular outcome. The individual could have several beliefs, but only some are available at any one time, and these readily available beliefs determine the prevailing attitude toward a behaviour.

Normative beliefs connote behavioural expectations of referent individuals as spouse, family, friends, doctor, teacher, and so on. These normative beliefs, combined with a person's motivation to adhere to the different referents, determine the prevailing subjective norm.

Control beliefs signify the prevalence of factors that could impede or advance behavioural performance. These control beliefs combined with

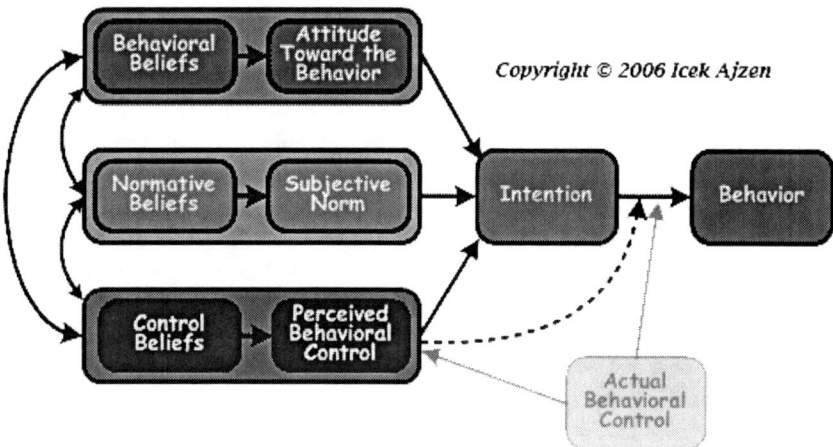

Figure 2.1 The theory of planned behaviour

the power of each control factor determine the prevailing perceived behavioural control.

Ajzen (2012) recently summarized the three concerns that direct human behaviour thusly: that intention is the direct antecedent of behaviour, which is also a function of attitude toward that behaviour, subjective norm and perceived behavioural control; that these determinants emanate, respectively, from beliefs concerning the possible consequences of the behaviour, the normative expectations of people who are significant and the prevalence of factors that control the behaviour. He noted that many correlational studies have verified the capacity of TPB to predict intentions and behaviour, in that changes in behavioural, normative and control beliefs can generate changes in intentions, and it is these changes in intentions that are reproduced in subsequent behaviours. Ajzen (2011) argued that the foundation of TPB is to predict intentions, and whether intentions predict behaviour is not only within the realm of the individual, but also in the dominion of others who exert actual control over that behaviour. However, Ajzen also explained that the more favourable the attitude and subjective norm, and the larger the perceived control, the greater the person's intention to effect the behaviour (2011). Armitage and Conner (2001) conducted a systematic review of 185 studies on TPB and found it to be efficacious for predicting intentions and behaviour. Perceived behavioural control, one of the constructs of TPB, on its own, predicted intentions and behaviour in several domains. This meta-analysis showed that measures of intention, self-prediction and desires have discriminant validity. Even so, in the event that a behaviour becomes problematic to achieve, then there is need to combine perceived behavioural control with intention (Ajzen 2002).

Nonetheless, the literature review in this book shows that notwithstanding good to moderate knowledge of HIV and AIDS among high school students, they still produced behaviours that harboured myths and misconceptions about HIV and AIDS (some examples are: DiClemente, Zorn and Temoshok 1986; Dias et al. 2006; DiClemente et al. 1988; Tavoosi et al. 2004; Yazdi et al. 2006; Pattullo et al. 1994; Agrawal et al. 1999; Hancock et al. 1999; Mahat and Scoloveno 2006; Norman, Carr and Jiménez 2006).

There were also findings on low HIV and AIDS knowledge (some examples are: Iryani et al. 2009; McManus and Dhar 2008; Pramanik et al. 2006; Di Clemente et al. 1986; Macchi et al. 2008; Bankhole et al. 2007); and studies that showed students with inappropriate attitudes toward PLHIV, HIV and AIDS (some examples are: Yazdi et al. 2006; Tavoosi et al. 2004; Movahed and Shoaa 2010; Yoo et al. 2005; Pattullo et al. 1994; Mahat and Scoloveno 2006; Odusanya and Bankole 2006; Norman, Carr and Jimenez 2006),

In these situations, planned or appropriate behaviours were not achieved. Ajzen's theory of planned behaviour would posit that the high school students' attitudes toward the desired behaviours, their subjective norms and their perceptions of behavioural control did not flow from their behavioural, normative and control beliefs. Notwithstanding whether these beliefs were "inaccurate, biased or otherwise irrational, our beliefs produce attitudes, intentions, and behaviours consistent with these beliefs" (Geraerts et al. 2008). These students' behaviours were not planned or reasoned because their intentions were not yet formed, and for this reason, they were not yet ready to engage in the desired behaviours. Ajzen (2011) argues that "behavioral intentions are indications of a person's readiness to perform a behavior".

Chapter 3

Methodology

Research Design

This study comprised fifteen secondary schools, coeducational and religious, with a total population of 2,911 students in one county of Guyana. The aims of this study are (1) to survey the HIV and AIDS knowledge, attitudes and beliefs of high school students; (2) to identify differences in knowledge and attitudes/perceptions by gender, age, ethnicity and religious groups; (3) to determine the relationship between HIV and AIDS knowledge and stigma-related attitudes/perceptions; and (4) to ascertain the predictors of both HIV and AIDS knowledge and HIV and AIDS stigma-related attitudes/perceptions.

This cross-sectional study was conducted to measure HIV and AIDS knowledge and stigma-related attitudes among high school students in Guyana who are the population of interest. A cross-sectional design does have the capacity to test relationships between variables and to generate hypotheses. For instance, a cross-sectional study (Dumitrescu et al. 2011) among first-year medical students tested the theory of planned behaviour to improve oral health behaviours. The study assessed intentions, attitudes, subjective norms, perceived behavioural control, oral health knowledge and current oral hygiene behaviours and did show that attitude, perceived behavioural control and oral health knowledge can predict intention to enhance oral health behaviours. The literature review for this study has numerous examples of cross-sectional studies testing relationships between variables.

The survey method was the preferred mode of observation because individual students constituted the unit of analysis, and because the survey method is an appropriate medium for measuring attitudes and beliefs in a huge population of students. A self-administered survey was conducted because of the sensitive nature of HIV data, and because of the fact that the survey method would preserve the anonymity of the participants (Babbie 1995).

Participants and Procedures

The sample of 379 students reflects the national characteristics. The national demographics in 2002 were: Indians: 43.5%; Africans: 30.2%; Mixed: 16.7%; Amerindians: 9.2%; Chinese: 0.19%; and Portuguese: 0.2%. Religious groups: Christians: 57.4%; Hindus: 28.4%; Muslims: 7.3%; Other: 1.3%. In the total population, the 13–18 age group constitutes about 20%.

Participants were selected on the basis of a purposive sample of 379 (218 females and 161 males) Guyanese high school students. Participants were within the 13–18 age group, with students from Form 3 (Grade 10) through Form 6 (Grade 12). These students belonged to various religious groups and ethnic backgrounds. Of the sample, 202 (53%) were Christians, 88 (23%) were Hindus, 37 (10%) were Muslims and 52 (14%) were members of other religious groups (non-Christian, non-Hindu and non-Muslim). Additionally, 154 (40%) were of African descent, 146 (38%) were of Indian descent, 6 (2%) were of Chinese descent, 15 (4%) were of Amerindian descent, 10 (3%) were of Portuguese descent and 48 (13%) were of mixed races (or Mixed). Area sampling was utilized to select students from Regions 3, 4 and 10 to secure geographical distribution of participants. These regions were selected because of the variance in the range of HIV prevalence as follows: Region 3 (10.62%), Region 4 (56.29%) and Region 10 (3.06%).

The sample of 379 students was selected from these fifteen high schools (thirteen government and two private):

Table 3.1 Participants by School

Schools	Number of Participants	Forms 3–6 Population
HS 1	19	271
HS 2	29	225
HS 3	20	262
HS 4	20	174
HS 5	61	78
HS 6	20	190
HS 7	20	167
HS 8	20	198
HS 9	20	115

Table 3.1 Participants by School (continued)

Schools	Number of Participants	Forms 3–6 Population
HS 10	37	177
HS 11	19	142
HS 12	19	298
HS 13	20	200
HS 14	20	209
HS 15	35	205
Total (N)	379	2911

Instruments

HIV and AIDS knowledge

HIV and AIDS knowledge was assessed utilizing the AIDS 101 Quiz from the Business Responds to AIDS/Labor Responds to AIDS (BRTA/LRTA) of the Centers for Disease Control and Prevention (CDC) – refer to http://Hivatwork.org/tools/quiz_a.htm. This quiz was used in national workshops by this author to develop Guyana's National HIV and AIDS Workplace Policy, and was selected because it includes seven standard dimensions of HIV and AIDS knowledge – impact of HIV and AIDS, symptoms of HIV and AIDS, myths and misconceptions of HIV transmission, clinical modes of HIV transmission, HIV testing, blood donation, and preventative measures. The ten-item questionnaire was modified in relation to the cultural context in Guyana. Cronbach's alpha coefficient was used to measure the internal consistency of the ten items on knowledge, and it yielded a satisfactory result of 0.72. Many businesses and labour unions in the US use this knowledge quiz.

The items were scored on the basis of "Correct" and "Incorrect" and participants were required to select a response. Based on the responses given, participants were categorized into three groups: the "Good Knowledge" group (those scoring > 90%), the "Moderate Knowledge" group (those scoring 75% but < 90%) and the "Poor Knowledge" group (those scoring ≤ 75%). The mean of the data distribution (74.5%) was applied as the basis for this determination.

The main variables were HIV and AIDS knowledge and attitudes, and intermediary demographic variables. According to Uutela (1976), attitude comprises three components: cognitive (knowledge), affective (feelings) and action (behaviour). Huskinson and Haddock (2004) found that persons with affective attitudes may be influenced by affect-type information, while those with cognitive attitudes may be influenced by cognitive information. Therefore, on this basis, HIV prevention interventions would have

Table 3.2 Knowledge of HIV and AIDS Questionnaire

1. AIDS is a disease that weakens the human body's immune system, making it difficult to fight infections and exposing persons infected to a number of serious, often fatal illnesses. (*True*)
2. Loss of appetite, weight loss, fever, night sweats, skin rashes, diarrhoea, tiredness, lack of resistance to infection or swollen lymph nodes are signs and symptoms of AIDS or other AIDS-related conditions. (*True*)
3. HIV is spread from an infected person to a non-infected person through casual physical contact – such as hugging, handshaking, traveling in the same vehicle, touching the same papers, or sharing the same office furniture, telephone or computer. (*False*)
4. HIV is spread through unprotected sexual intercourse (vaginal, anal or oral sex) with infected persons, use or sharing of contaminated needles with infected persons, mother-to-child transmissions during pregnancy or childbirth, and sometimes through transfusions or other exchanges of HIV-infected blood. (*True*)
5. HIV cannot be transmitted by sneezing, coughing, or by using sinks, bathrooms, toilets, eating or drinking utensils used by an infected person, or by eating food prepared by an infected person. (*True*)
6. If a person is tested positive for HIV when he/she takes the antibody test, it does not mean that the person has AIDS. In fact, a person who has AIDS may show no signs or symptoms of the disease and may not develop AIDS for many years. (*True*)
7. A blood donor cannot get HIV while giving blood. (*True*)
8. A person can get HIV from animals (such as cats and dogs) around the home and from mosquitoes. (*False*)
9. A person is likely to contract HIV by being around or working with an infected person on a daily basis and over a long period of time. (*False*)
10. To protect yourself and/or those you work with from being infected with HIV, you will need to take or put into place preventative measures. (*True*).

to present the appropriate type of information in order to influence individual's attitudes/perceptions of HIV, AIDS and PLHIV.

Stigma-related attitudes/perceptions

Stigma-related attitudes/perceptions were assessed using the Horizon/Population Council (Stewart, Pulerwitz and Esu-Wiliams 2002) with cultural modifications for Guyana. The stigma-related attitude thirteen item scale (see table 3.3) has eight dimensions of beliefs: HIV and AIDS as death, as punishment, as crime, as horror, as derision, as social exclusion and marginalization, as social labelling and stereotyping, and being insus-

Table 3.3 HIV and AIDS Stigma-related Attitudes/Perceptions

1. HIV and AIDS is death.
2. HIV and AIDS is punishment.
3. HIV and AIDS is a crime.
4. HIV and AIDS only happen to others, not me.
5. HIV and AIDS is horror.
6. "People make jokes about people who are HIV-positive." (*False*)
7. "If I had AIDS, people would call me names and gossip about me." (*False*)
8. People with HIV or AIDS should not be permitted to work. (*False*)
9. People with HIV or AIDS should not sell food. (*False*)
10. Not comfortable holding hands with a person who is HIV-positive. (*False*)
11. Not comfortable sharing work tools with an HIV- or AIDS-infected person. (*False*)
12. Not comfortable sharing the same toilet as a person with HIV or AIDS. (*False*)
13. If a person is seen sitting next to an HIV- or AIDS-positive person, people might think that that person also has HIV or AIDS. (*False*)

ceptible to HIV and AIDS. Cronbach's alpha coefficient was used to measure the internal consistency of the thirteen items on stigma-related attitudes and yielded a score of 0.56.

The items were scored on the basis of "Appropriate" and "Inappropriate", and participants were required to select a response. Based on the responses given, participants were categorized into two groups: the "Appropriate" group (those scoring > 75%) and the "Not Appropriate" group (those scoring ≤ 75%).

Intermediary Variables

The following intermediary variables were used:

- Sex: male/female
- Age groups: 13–15; 16–18.
- Religious groups: Christian, Hindu, Islam, Other (non-Christian, non-Hindu, non-Islam)
- Ethnic groups: African, Indian, Chinese, Amerindian, Portuguese, Mixed

The questionnaire elicited responses on demographic variables of sex, age, religious groups and ethnicity in order to provide an appropriate description of the sample, to identify any relationship between the demographics and

HIV and AIDS knowledge, and demographics and HIV and AIDS stigma-related attitudes/perceptions.

Data Collection

The study utilized a self-administered questionnaire with closed-ended responses that sought answers from 379 high school students of both sexes. These students, who were between the ages of 13 and 18 and who were Forms 3 to 6, were from both rural and urban neighbourhoods. Teachers from the classrooms administered the questionnaires to the students and also retrieved the completed questionnaires.

Data Analysis

The Statistical Package for the Social Sciences (SPSS), Version 16.0 and StatsDirect facilitated the processing and analysis of the questionnaire data. Descriptive statistics were used to measure the demographics and individual item scores on knowledge and attitudes/perceptions. The independent samples t-test was employed to determine the differences in HIV and AIDS knowledge between the genders and among the different age groups. The Kruskal-Wallis (K-W) was used to ascertain the differences in HIV and AIDS knowledge among the various religious and ethnic groups. The independent samples t-test was also used to determine the differences in stigma-related attitudes/perceptions between gender and age. Analysis of variance (ANOVA) was used to measure the differences in stigma-related attitudes/perceptions among the different religious persuasions. The K-W was applied to determine the differences in stigma-related attitudes/perceptions among the different ethnic groups. Finally, the logistic regression model was employed to identify confounders, and to determine the factors that influence HIV and AIDS knowledge development and stigma-related attitudes/perceptions. The tests used a significance level of $p < 0.05$.

Ethical Considerations

The Ministry of Education issued permission to conduct the study. Each principal (or their respective representatives) was contacted personally and through a letter that explained the scope and benefits of the study and participants' rights. The letter also sought consent from students to participate in the study. This letter was attached to the questionnaire. This approach is consistent with the Nuremberg Code of 1947 which requires that the human subject voluntarily consents to participate in the study. Participants were also informed of the purpose, procedure, inconvenience and likely hazards of the study.

Chapter 4

HIV and AIDS Knowledge

Descriptive Statistics – Knowledge and Demographics

This study, conducted in 2009–2010, contains questionnaire data from 379 diverse students between the ages of 13 and 18 years old. The 19-and-over age group was removed from the data set, as it constituted less than 1% (or 2 persons) in the sample.

Table 4.1 Demographic Characteristics

Characteristics	N (379)	Per Cent Total
Male	161	42
Female	218	58
Religious Group		
Christian	202	53
Hindu	88	23
Muslim	37	10
Other	52	14
Ethnic Group/Ethnicity		
African	154	40
Indian	146	38
Chinese	6	2
Amerindian	15	4
Portuguese	10	3
Mixed	48	13
Age Group		
13–15	148	39
16–18	229	60

The majority of the students surveyed were females (58%), and over half of the sample comprised the senior group (60%). Additionally, the greater part of the sample consisted of Africans and Indians (78%), and a little over half of the number of students surveyed were Christians (53%).

This section depicts the Guyana high school students' understanding of both the normative and non-normative (myths and misconceptions) aspects of HIV and AIDS. Normative aspects of HIV and AIDS pertain to the scientifically accepted knowledge (an example is: AIDS is a disease that weakens the human body's immune system, making it difficult to fight infections and exposing persons infected to a number of serious, often fatal illnesses.). Non-normative aspects of HIV and AIDS relate to misconceptions and myths surrounding HIV and AIDS (an example is: HIV is spread from an infected person to a non-infected person through casual physical contact – such as hugging, handshaking, travelling in the same vehicle, touching the same papers, or sharing the same office furniture, telephone or computer.).

Table 4.2 shows that students have moderate knowledge of HIV and AIDS. But are students' understandings of the normative and non-normative aspects of HIV and AIDS normally distributed? Are these extreme observations? These answers lie in determining whether the observations on HIV and AIDS knowledge are normally distributed by means of a histogram, the normal probability plot and descriptive statistics. Establishing the status of the distribution would determine the types of statistical procedure to be used for analysis of the data.

Figure 4.1 shows that the histogram with an almost bell-shaped appearance seems to be normally distributed. The Q-Q plot shows the data on a straight line and, therefore, the data is normally distributed (figure 4.2).

The mean and median are fairly similar: 7.47 and 8.00, respectively. The range is 8.00. These indicators suggest that the data are normally distributed.

Table 4.3 shows that high school students in Guyana have moderate knowledge of HIV and AIDS. The students scored correctly on an average of 7.47 out of 10 statements, just over half of the students (55.9%) responded incorrectly to only one statement and they possess this level of knowledge without exposure to any formal school curriculum on HIV and AIDS education. Nearly all the Guyana students in the sample fully understand the modes of HIV transmission; 97.4% correctly responded to this statement: "HIV is spread through unprotected sexual intercourse (vaginal, anal or oral sex) with infected persons, use or sharing of contaminated needles with infected persons, mother-to-child transmission during pregnancy or childbirth and sometimes through transfusions or other exchanges of HIV-infected blood." Most of the Guyanese high school students recognized the signs and symptoms of HIV and AIDS;

Table 4.2 Knowledge of HIV and AIDS

	Frequency		Per Cent Total	
Variables (Questions)	**Correct**	**Not Correct**	**Correct**	**Not Correct**
1. AIDS is a disease that weakens the human body's immune system, making it difficult to fight infections and exposing persons infected to a number of serious, often fatal illnesses. (*True*)	350	29	92.3	7.7
2. Loss of appetite, weight loss, fever, night sweats, skin rashes, diarrhoea, tiredness, lack of resistance to infection or swollen lymph nodes are signs and symptoms of AIDS or other AIDS-related conditions. (*True*)	357	22	94.2	5.8
3. HIV is spread from an infected person to a non-infected person through casual physical contact – such as hugging, handshaking, travelling in the same vehicle, touching the same papers, or sharing the same office furniture, telephone or computer. (*False*)	317	62	83.6	16.4
4. HIV is spread through unprotected sexual intercourse (vaginal, anal or oral sex) with infected persons, use or sharing of contaminated needles with infected persons, mother-to-child transmissions during pregnancy or childbirth, and sometimes through transfusions or other exchanges of HIV-infected blood. (*True*)	369	10	97.4	2.6
5. HIV cannot be transmitted by sneezing, coughing, or by using sinks, bathrooms, toilets, eating or drinking utensils used by an infected person, or by eating food prepared by an infected person. (*True*)	308	71	81.3	18.7

Table 4.2 Knowledge of HIV and AIDS (continued)

Variables (Questions)	Frequency		Per Cent Total	
	Correct	Not Correct	Correct	Not Correct
6. If a person is tested positive for HIV when he/she takes the antibody test, it does not mean that the person has AIDS. In fact, a person who has AIDS may show no signs or symptoms of the disease and may not develop AIDS for many years. (*True*)	315	64	83.1	16.9
7. A blood donor cannot get HIV while giving blood. (*True*)	167	212	44.1	55.9
8. A person can get HIV from animals (such as cats and dogs) around the home and from mosquitoes. (*False*)	307	72	81.0	19.0
9. A person is likely to contract HIV by being around or working with an infected person on a daily basis and over a long period of time. (*False*)	316	63	83.4	16.6
10. To protect yourself and/or those you work with from being infected with HIV, you will need to take or put into place preventative measures. (*True*)	265	114	69.9	30.1

94.2% correctly responded to the statement: "Loss of appetite, weight loss, fever, night sweats, skin rashes, diarrhoea, tiredness, lack of resistance to infection or swollen lymph nodes are signs and symptoms of AIDS or other AIDS-related conditions"; and 92.3% know that "AIDS is a disease that weakens the human body's immune system, making it difficult to fight infections and exposing persons infected to a number of serious, often fatal illnesses."

Interestingly, fewer than half of the Guyanese students surveyed supported the view that a blood donor cannot get HIV while giving blood. In Guyana, high school students still express concerns about contagion, notwithstanding their moderate HIV knowledge of the transmission modes. In this case, knowledge does not have an impact on attitude and behaviour change.

In addition, about 20% (or one-fifth) of high school students in Guyana viewed the following as modes of HIV transmission: casual physical contact;

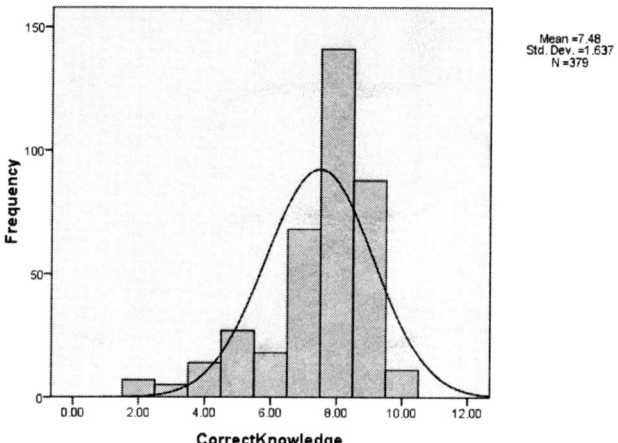

Figure 4.1 Knowledge of HIV and AIDS – histogram

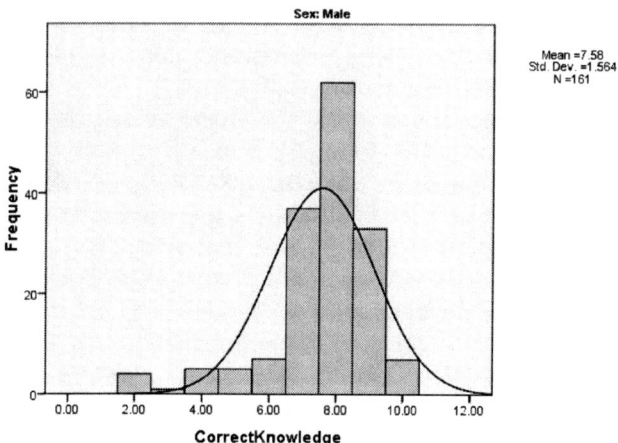

Figure 4.2 Knowledge of HIV and AIDS (males)

Table 4.3 Descriptive Statistics for Overall Correct Knowledge

Correct Knowledge Descriptives	Value
Valid	379.000
Missing	.000
Mean	7.478
Std. Error of Mean	.084
Median	8.000
Mode	8.000
Std. Deviation	1.637
Variance	2.679
Skewness	−1.308
Std. Error of Skewness	.125
Kurtosis	1.619
Std. Error of Kurtosis	.250
Range	8.000
Minimum	2.000
Maximum	10.000
Sum	2834.000

sneezing; coughing; using sinks, bathrooms and toilets used by PLHIV; being around cats and dogs; being bitten by mosquitoes; and being around people at the workplace over a protracted period.

Kendall's W evaluates respondents' agreement among their rankings of HIV and AIDS knowledge, and Kendall's W at .477 shows that respondents showed good agreement on their rankings. Since the calculated p-value is 0.000, which is less than $\alpha = 0.05$, then it is appropriate to conclude that Kendall's W is statistically significant, and, therefore, there are significant differences among the rankings for HIV and AIDS knowledge. With respect to levels of importance, students ranked knowledge of HIV transmission modes (item 4) as the most important, the knowledge of the symptoms of AIDS and AIDS-related illnesses (item 2) as the second most important, and the knowledge of the effects of HIV and AIDS on the immune system (item 1) as the third most important. Students viewed the other seven items as having lesser importance.

Table 4.4 Kendall's W Test of the Knowledge Items Ranks

Item	Mean Rank	Rank
Weaken immune system	7.05	3
AIDS symptoms	7.14	2
Casual physical contact	3.25	10
Transmission methods	7.30	1
Non-transmission methods	6.49	5
AIDS status	6.58	4
Blood donor risk	4.63	7
Human/animal transmission	3.38	8
Working with people with HIV	3.26	9
Preventative measure	5.92	6

Table 4.5 Kendall's W Test Significance for Knowledge Items

Test Statistics

N	379.000
Kendall's W^a	.477
Chi-Square	1627.318
Df	9.000
Asymp. Sig.	.000

a. Kendall's Coefficient of Concordance

Knowledge and Demographics

The next part of this chapter presents the following tests of hypotheses about population means for HIV and AIDS knowledge and the demographics of gender, age, religion and ethnicity:

- There are no differences in the mean scores for HIV and AIDS knowledge between male and female high school students.
- There are no differences in the mean scores for HIV and AIDS knowledge among the different age groups of high school students.
- There are no differences in the mean scores for HIV and AIDS knowledge among the religious groups of high school students.
- There are no differences in the mean scores for HIV and AIDS knowledge among the different ethnic groups of high school students.

Sex

Female (60.1%) and male (56.5%) high school students in Guyana have fair knowledge of HIV and AIDS. The differences in knowledge scores between male and female high school students were tested with the use of the independent sample t-test, since the dependent variable (HIV and AIDS knowledge) observations are numeric and the explanatory variable (sex) is dichotomous; the hypotheses are:

- $H_0{:}\mu_1 = \mu_2$ There are no differences in the mean scores for HIV and AIDS knowledge between male and female high school students. (Null Hypothesis)
- $H_1{:}\mu_1 \neq \mu_2$ There are differences in the mean scores for HIV and AIDS knowledge between male and female high school students. (Alternative Hypothesis)
- μ_1: refers to similar mean scores for HIV and AIDS knowledge for male and female high school students.
- μ_2: refers to different mean scores for HIV and AIDS knowledge for male and female high school students.

The assumptions for the independent samples t-test are as follows:

1. The samples are independent.
2. The observations in each sample are independent.
3. The variances are similar.
4. The data are normally distributed.

Assumptions 1 and 2 are part of the study design, and for this reason, these assumptions are satisfied. The histogram, the normal probability plot and descriptive statistics were used to determine whether the data for HIV and AIDS knowledge among the two genders are normally distributed.

The histograms and the normal probability plots for HIV and AIDS knowledge among the sexes show that the data are normally distributed. Table 4.6 shows that the mean and median for both males and females are 7.58 and 7.40, and 8.00 and 8.00, respectively. Assumption 4, therefore, is satisfied.

We can assume that the variances for male and female high school students are similar at 2.45 and 2.85, respectively. Therefore, assumption 3 is satisfied. Clearly, then, the assumptions for conducting an unpaired t-test are satisfied.

The comparison of the variances shows that we need to assume equal variances. The t-test provides a t-statistic = 1.023 and a p-value = 0.307, which is greater than 0.05 (table 4.7). There is, therefore, no evidence to reject the null hypothesis. The conclusion can be made that, overall, there is no significant difference in the mean scores for HIV and AIDS knowledge between male and female high school students.

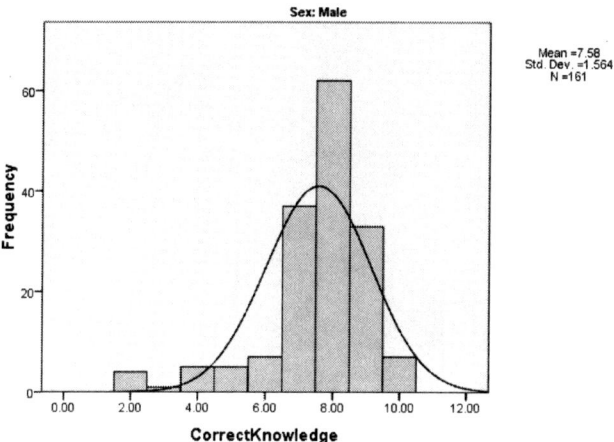

Figure 4.3 Correct knowedge of HIV and AIDS (males) – histogram

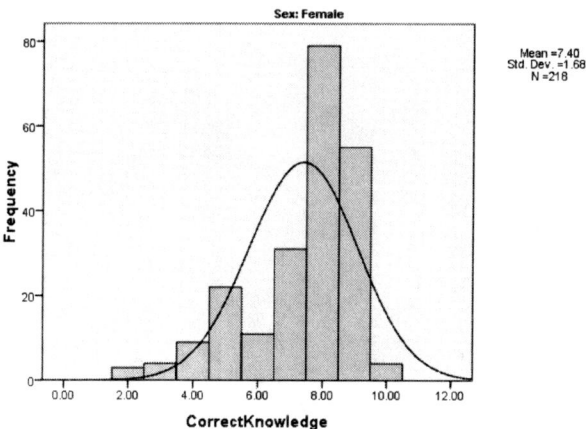

Figure 4.4 Correct knowedge of HIV and AIDS (females) – histogram

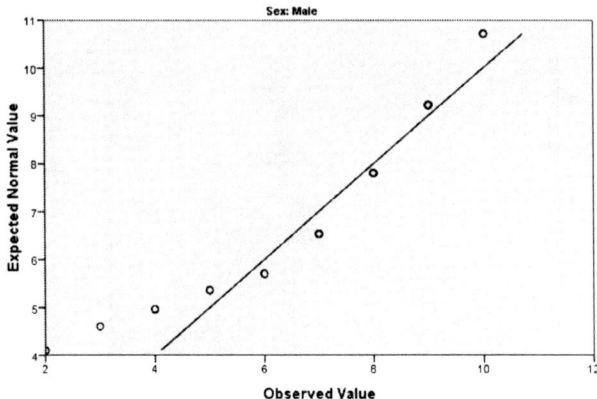

Figure 4.5 Correct knowedge of HIV and AIDS (males) – normal Q-Q
plot

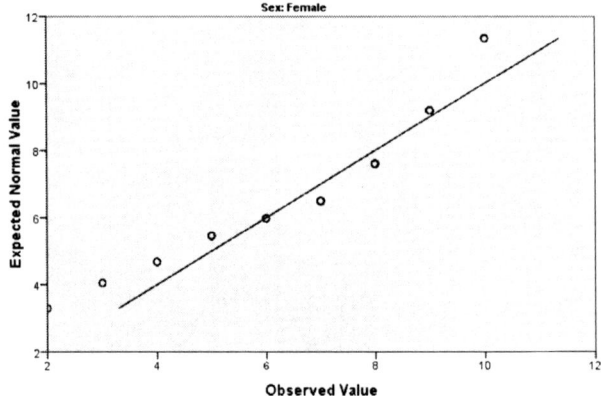

Figure 4.6 Correct knowedge of HIV and AIDS (females) – normal Q-
Q plot

Table 4.6 Descriptive Statistics for Correct Knowledge (Sex)

Descriptives	Male	Female
Valid	161.00	218.00
Missing	.00	.00
Mean	7.58	7.40
Std. Error of Mean	.12	.11
Median	8.00	8.00
Mode	8.00	8.00
Std. Deviation	1.56	1.69
Variance	2.45	2.85
Range	8.00	8.00
Minimum	2.00	2.00
Maximum	10.00	10.00
Sum	1220.00	1614.00

Male and female high school students showed no differences in their HIV and AIDS knowledge scores on most of the knowledge items (see appendix 1). A huge proportion of both genders (91.3% of the females and 94% of the males) recognized that AIDS is a disease that impairs the human body's immune system, making it tough to battle infections and exposing persons infected to a number of serious, often fatal illnesses. High school students (96.3% females and 91.3% males) believe that loss of appetite, weight loss, fever, night sweats, skin rashes, diarrhoea, tiredness, lack of resistance to infection or swollen lymph nodes are signs and symptoms of AIDS or other AIDS-related conditions. Some 98% females and 97% males knew that HIV transmission happens through unprotected sexual intercourse (vaginal, anal or oral sex) with HIV-infected persons, sharing contaminated needles with HIV-infected persons, mother-to-child transmissions during pregnancy or childbirth, and occasionally through transfusions or other contacts with HIV-infected blood.

Both sexes were aware that should a person test positive for HIV when that person takes the antibody test, it does not indicate that that person has AIDS. These students (83% females and 82.2% males) were aware, too, that an AIDS-infected person may manifest no disease symptoms or signs, and may take some time to reach the onset of AIDS. Given that students only showed moderate knowledge of HIV and AIDS, it is hardly surprising that they (80.3% females and 82% males) would believe that a person can contract HIV from having animals (such as cats and dogs) around the home and from mosquitoes. Students who believed that prevention measures were necessary as a protection from an HIV-infected person at the workplace comprised only 71.1% females and 68.3% males. These results suggest that sex has no impact on HIV and AIDS knowledge.

Table 4.7 Group Statistics: Unpaired t-test for Gender and Knowledge

	Gender	N	Mean	Std. Deviation	Std. Error Mean
Correct Knowledge	Male	161	7.5776	1.56381	.12325
	Female	218	7.4037	1.68823	.11434

Independent Sample Test

		Levene's Test for Equality of Variances		t-test for Equality of Means					95% Confidence Interval of the Difference	
		F	Sig.	t	Df	Sig. (2-tailed)	Mean Difference	Std. Error Difference	Lower	Upper
Correct Knowledge	Equal variances assumed	3.798	.052	1.023	377	.307	.17397	.17007	-.16043	.50837
	Equal variances not assumed			1.035	358.266	.301	.17397	.16812	-.15665	.50459

Source: StatsDirect

Age

Just over half (55.4%) of the 13–15 age group demonstrated moderate knowledge and just under half (44.6%) demonstrated poor knowledge of HIV and AIDS. About two-thirds (68.6%) of the 16–18 age group showed moderate knowledge, and about a third (31.4%) showed poor knowledge of HIV and AIDS. The differences in knowledge among the different age groups (13–15 and 16–18) of high school students were tested with the use of the independent sample t-test, since the dependent variable (knowledge) observations are numeric and the explanatory variable (age) is dichotomous; the hypotheses are:

- $H_0:\mu_1 = \mu_2$ There are no differences in the mean scores for HIV and AIDS knowledge between the two age groups of high school students. (Null Hypothesis)
- $H_1:\mu_1 \neq \mu_2$ There are differences in the mean scores for HIV and AIDS knowledge between the two age groups of high school students. (Alternative Hypothesis)
- μ_1: refers to similar mean scores for HIV and AIDS knowledge between the different age groups of high school students.
- μ_2: refers to different mean scores for HIV and AIDS knowledge between the different age groups of high school students.

Mention has already been made on the assumptions of the t-test (refer to section titled "Gender"). Assumptions 1 and 2 are implicit in the study design, and for this reason, these assumptions are satisfied.

The histograms for HIV and AIDS knowledge among both age groups are normally distributed, and the normal probability plots for HIV and AIDS knowledge among both age groups approximate a straight line. Table 4.7 shows that the means and medians for both age groups are fairly similar. We can, therefore, assume that the observations for both age groups are normally distributed.

The variances may be regarded as unequal at 3.58 and 2.05. Nonetheless, whether we proceed with the t-test, or its non-parametric equivalent, the Mann-Whitney test, depends on whether the data are normally distributed. The histograms, the normal probability plots and descriptive statistics show that the data are normally distributed, so the t-test will be performed.

Overall, table 4.9 shows the t-test provides a t-statistic = –2.520 and a p-value of p = 0.018, which is smaller than p = 0.05. There is evidence then to reject the null hypothesis. It can therefore be concluded that there are statistically significant differences ($p < 0.05$) in the mean level of HIV and AIDS knowledge between the 13–15 and the 16–18 age groups of high school students in the Guyana sample.

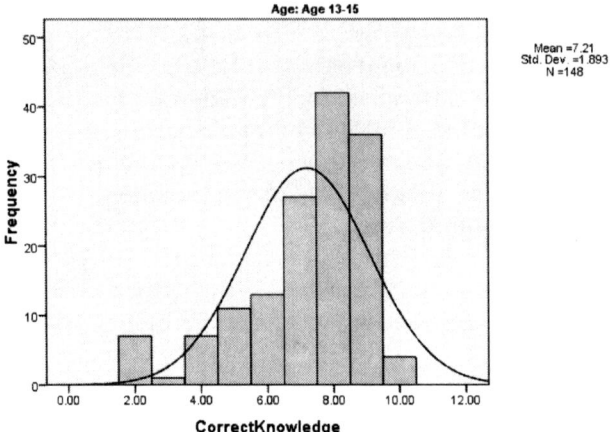

Figure 4.7 Correct knowedge of HIV and AIDS (age 13–15) – histogram

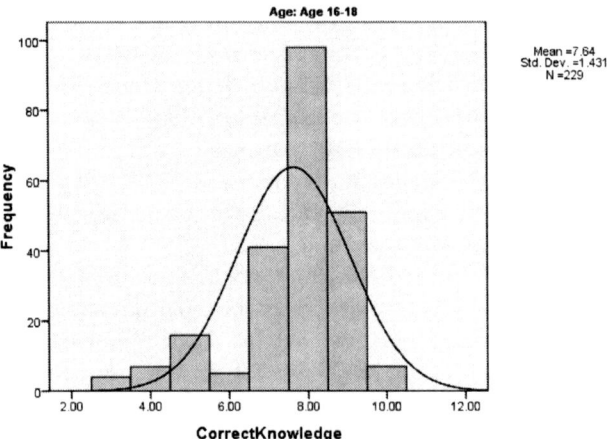

Figure 4.8 Correct knowedge of HIV and AIDS (age 16–18) – histogram

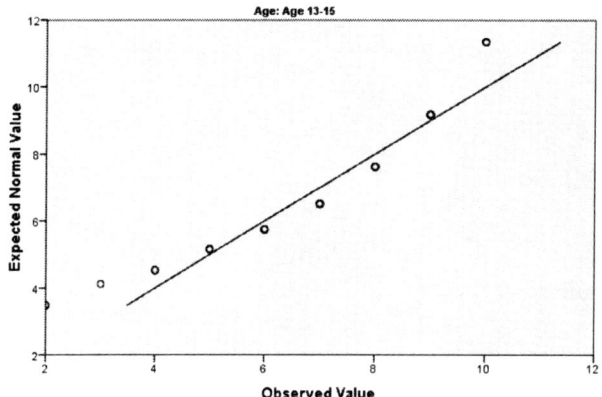

Figure 4.9 Correct knowedge of HIV and AIDS (age 13–15) – normal Q-Q plot

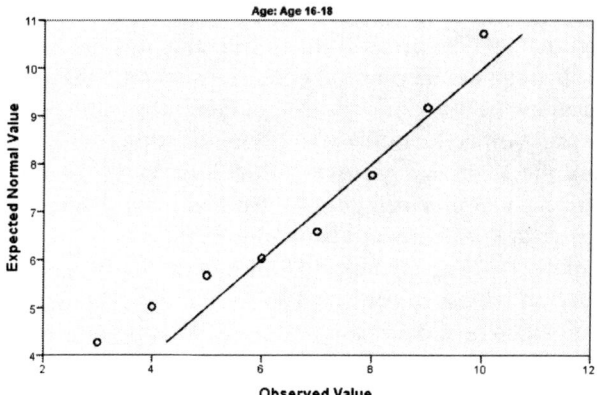

Figure 4.10 Correct knowedge of HIV and AIDS (age 16–18) – normal Q-Q plot

Table 4.8 Descriptive Statistics: Age

	Age Groups	
	Age 13–15	**Age 16–18**
Valid	148.00	229.00
Missing	.00	.00
Mean	7.21	7.64
Std. Error of Mean	.16	.09
Median	8.00	8.00
Mode	8.00	8.00
Std. Deviation	1.89	1.43
Variance	3.58	2.05
Range	8.00	7.00
Minimum	2.00	3.00
Maximum	10.00	10.00
Sum	1067.00	1750.00

There are statistically significant differences ($p < 0.05$) in the mean HIV and AIDS knowledge of the 13–15 and 16–18 age groups of high school students on three aspects (see appendix 2):

1. 75.7% of the 13–15 age group and 88.6% of the 16–18 age group believed that HIV is spread from an infected person to a non-infected person through casual physical contact – such as hugging, handshaking, travelling in the same vehicle, touching the same papers, or sharing the same office furniture, telephone or computer.
2. 71.6% of the 13–15 age group and 86.9% of the 16–18 age group believed that a person can get HIV from animals (such as cats and dogs) around the home and from mosquitoes.
3. 76.4% of the 13–15 age group and 87.8% of the 16–18 age group believed that a person is likely to contract HIV by being or working around an infected person on a daily basis and over a long period of time.

All three items are measures of myths and misconceptions about HIV. While both age groups showed moderate knowledge of the consequences of HIV on the immune system and the modes of transmission, there were differences in their knowledge about misconceptions and myths about HIV. In fact, the older age group more than the younger age group internalized the misconceptions and myths; the younger age group eventually could accept these myths and misconceptions, depending on the effectiveness of the older age group's peer influences.

Table 4.9 Group Statistics: Unpaired t-test for Age and Knowledge

	Age	N	Mean	Std. Deviation	Std. Error Mean
Correct	Age 13–15	148	7.2095	1.89253	.15557
Knowledge	Age 16–18	229	7.6419	1.43061	.09454

Independent Samples Test

		Levene's Test for Equality of Variances		t-test for Equality of Means					95% Confidence Interval of the Difference	
		F	Sig.	t	df	Sig. (2-tailed)	Mean Difference	Std. Error Difference	Lower	Upper
Correct Knowledge	Equal variances assumed	13.896	.000	-2.520	375	.012	-.43246	.17164	-.76995	-.09497
	Equal variances not assumed			-2.376	253.347	.018	-.43246	.18204	-.79096	-.07396

Source: StatsDirect

Religious Groups

The results showed that Christian (75.2%), Hindu (34%), Muslim (59.5%) and Other (71.2%) high school students have moderate HIV and AIDS knowledge. Differences in the mean scores for HIV and AIDS knowledge among high school students of different religious persuasions were tested; the hypotheses are:

- $H_0:\mu_1 = \mu_2$ There are no differences in the mean scores for HIV and AIDS knowledge among the different religious groups of high school students. (Null Hypothesis)
- $H_1:\mu_1 \neq \mu_2$ There are differences in the mean scores for HIV and AIDS knowledge among the different religious groups of high school students. (Alternative Hypothesis)
- μ_1: refers to similar mean scores for HIV and AIDS knowledge among the different religious groups of high school students.
- μ_2: refers to different mean scores for HIV and AIDS knowledge among the different religious groups of high school students.

Since there are more than two groups (Christians, Hindus, Muslims and Others), the t-test is not applicable. The ANOVA is the relevant statistical procedure to use, but first we have to determine whether its assumptions are satisfied. The assumptions of ANOVA are similar to those of a t-test, apart from the fact that there are more than two groups. The assumptions are as follows:

1. The groups are independent.
2. The observations in each group are independent.
3. The variances in each group are similar.
4. The observations in each group are normally distributed.

Assumptions 1 and 2 are part of the study design; therefore, we have to assume that they are satisfied. Histograms, normal probability plots and descriptive statistics were used to test these assumptions.

The histograms and the normal probability plots show that the data for the religious groups are normally distributed. The descriptive statistics show that the variances are different in each religious group: 0.986 (Christian), 4.310 (Hindu), 1.863 (Muslim) and 2.170 (Others)

Assumption 4 is satisfied while assumption 3 is not. The Levene F test (table 4.10) has a p-value of 0.000, and since it is less than p = 0.05, we.

Table 4.10 Levene F Test – Religious Groups

Levene Statistic	df1	df2	Sig.
33.446	3	375	.000

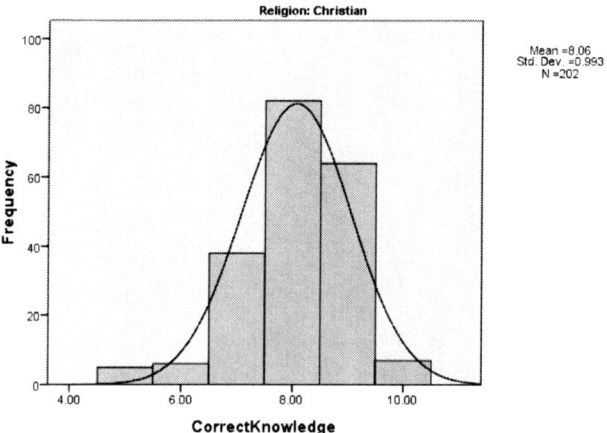

Figure 4.11 Correct knowedge of HIV and AIDS (Christians) –
    histogram

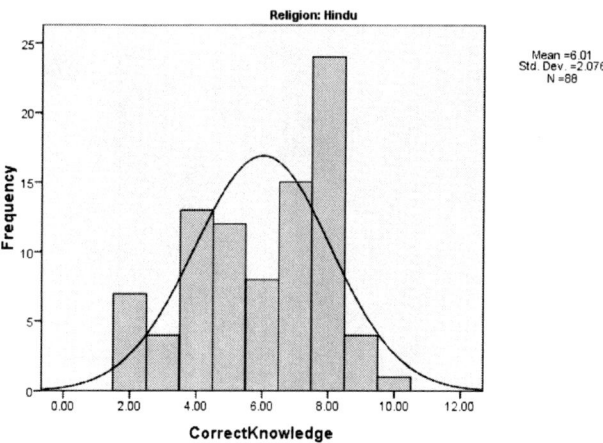

Figure 4.12 Correct knowedge of HIV and AIDS (Hindus) – histogram

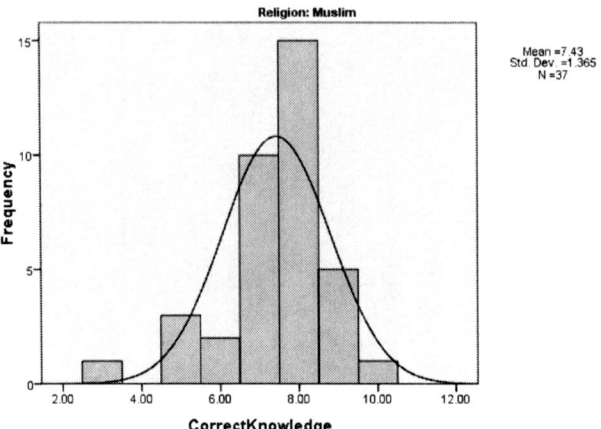

Figure 4.13 Correct knowedge of HIV and AIDS (Muslims) – histogram

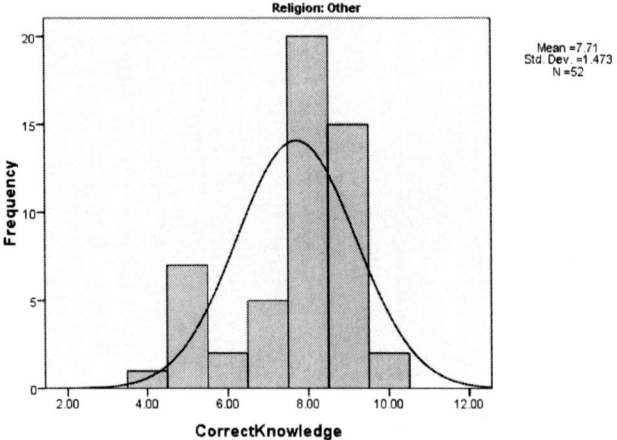

Figure 4.14 Correct knowedge of HIV and AIDS (other religious groups) – histogram

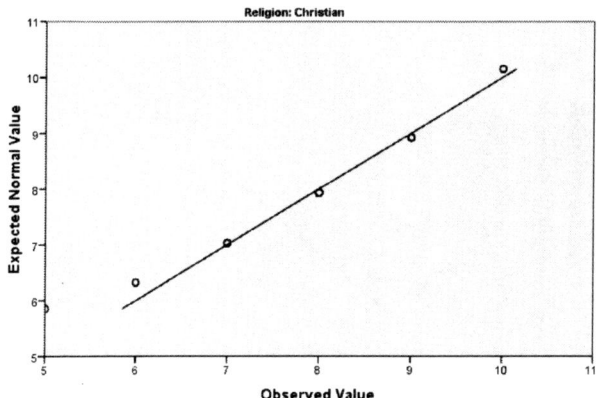

Figure 4.15 Correct knowedge of HIV and AIDS (Christians) – normal Q-Q plot

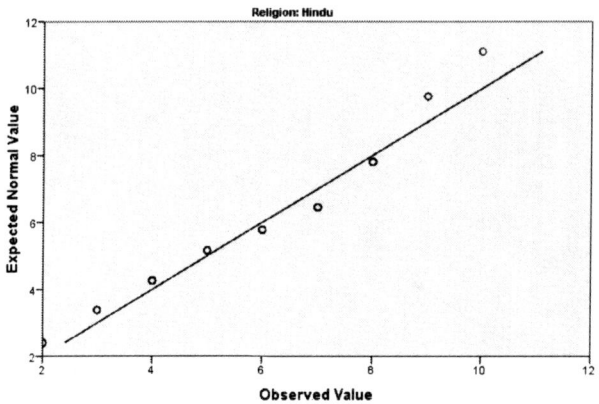

Figure 4.16 Correct knowedge of HIV and AIDS (Hindus) – normal Q-Q plot

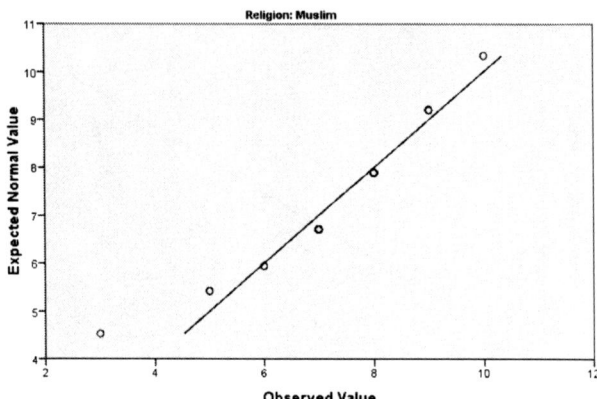

Figure 4.17 Correct knowedge of HIV and AIDS (Muslims) – normal Q-Q plot

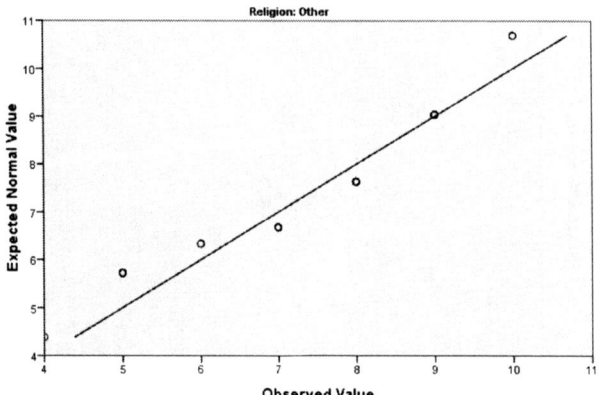

Figure 4.18 Correct knowedge of HIV and AIDS (other religious groups) – normal Q-Q plot

have evidence to reject the null hypothesis of no differences in variances. The variances, therefore, are not similar, and as such, the assumption that the variances have to be similar is not satisfied. The test showing no equality of variance indicates that we have to assume that there is variance in HIV and AIDS knowledge among the religious groups. We would, therefore, proceed to use the ANOVA's non-parametric equivalent, the Kruskal-Wallis (K-W) test.

The K-W test in table 4.11 shows that, overall, there is statistical significance in the median HIV and AIDS knowledge among the four religious groups of high school students. The K-W test results show p = 0.000. We can, therefore, reject the null hypothesis that there are no differences among these religious groups. We can now conclude that there are statistically significant differences (p < 0.05) in the median HIV and AIDS knowledge scores among students from different religious groups. The K-W test also identifies students by paired religious groups to demonstrate where the differences in median HIV and AIDS knowledge scores are likely to lie. The paired religious groups identified are: Christians and Muslims (p = 0.02), Christians and Hindus (p = 0.00), Muslims and Hindus (p = 0.00), and between other groups and Hindus (p = 0.00).

Table 4.11 Kruskal-Wallis Test Statistics and Pairwise Comparisons – Religious Groups

Variables: Total out of 10~Religious groups = 1,
   Total out of 10~Religious groups = 3,
   Total out of 10~Religious groups = 4,
   Total out of 10~Religious groups = 2

Groups = 4
  df = 3
  Total observations = 379

  T = 69.185501
  P < 0.0001

Adjusted for ties:
  T = 74.419521
  P < 0.0001

At least one of the sample populations tends to yield larger observations than at least one other sample population.

Kruskal-Wallis Significance Test – Religious Groups

Variables	Chi-square	df	Asymp. Sig
Question 1	44.561	3	.000
Question 2	.731	3	.866
Question 3	84.248	3	.000
Question 4	4.189	3	.242
Question 5	2.180	3	.536
Question 6	20.829	3	.000
Question 7	17.841	3	.000
Question 8	37.793	3	.000
Question 9	76.860	3	.000
Question 10	29.715	3	.000

**Kruskal-Wallis: All Pairwise Comparisons
(Dwass-Steel-Chritchlow-Fligner)**
Critical q (range) = 3.63316

Total out of 10~Religious groups = 1 vs. Total out of 10~Religious groups = 3	Significant
($|-4.046484| > 3.63316$)	P = 0.0219
Total out of 10~Religious groups = 1 vs. Total out of 10~Religious groups = 2	Significant
($|-11.901655| > 3.63316$)	P < 0.0001
Total out of 10~Religious groups = 3 vs. Total out of 10~Religious groups = 2	Significant
($|5.02933| > 3.63316$)	P = 0.0021
Total out of 10~Religious groups = 4 vs. Total out of 10~Religious groups = 2	Significant
($|7.141322| > 3.63316$)	P < 0.0001

Source: StatsDirect

In table 4.11, the K-W test also shows that there is a significant difference in median HIV and AIDS knowledge among students from different religious persuasions on seven out of ten items; therefore, the median "knowledge" scores emanate from different populations. Items 1, 3, 6, 7, 8, 9 and 10 represent the areas of difference of knowledge among students. These areas are as follows:

- AIDS is a disease that weakens the human immune system.
- HIV is spread by casual physical contact with infected persons.

- If a person tests positive for HIV, it does not follow that that person has AIDS.
- A blood donor cannot get HIV while giving blood.
- A person can contract HIV from animals at home or from mosquitoes.
- A person can contract HIV by being with an infected person.
- Protecting oneself as well as co-workers from contracting HIV would necessitate the use of preventive measures.

In table 4.12, the K-W test ranks as number one (items with the strongest difference) the following religious groups on each of the seven knowledge items that are statistically significant ($p < 0.05$):

- Christians indicated that AIDS is a disease that weakens the human immune system, and that it may be necessary to effect preventive measures for protection against contracting HIV;
- Hindus expressed scepticism with the scientifically accepted transmission modes vis-à-vis their belief that a person can contract HIV in the following ways: (1) through casual physical contact with infected persons, (2) from animals at home and from mosquitoes, and (3) by being with an infected person;
- Other groupings of high school students (no affiliation with Christianity, Hinduism or Islam) indicated that (1) if a person tests HIV-positive, it does not follow that that person has AIDS, and (2) that a blood donor cannot get HIV while giving blood.

The K-W test shows that we can reject the null hypothesis of no differences in median HIV and AIDS knowledge among students from various religious groups. In fact, there are differences in HIV and AIDS knowledge among the students with different religious persuasions. Table 4.12 provides the rankings of the mean scores for HIV and AIDS knowledge among the religious groups to depict areas of major differences. A high mean rank means a high score and a low mean rank denotes a low score. The K-W test results indicate that there are significant differences in median HIV and AIDS knowledge between these pairs ($p < 0.05$), as seen in table 4.13:

The following codes will be used to discuss the information presented in table 4.12:

- Christian students – Group C
- Hindu students – Group H
- Muslim students – Group M
- Other (students of other religious groups) – Group O

Table 4.12 Kruskal-Wallis (Ranks):
Religious Groups and Knowledge

Variables	Religious Groups	N	Mean Rank
Question 1	Christian	202	201.69
	Hindu	88	159.28
	Muslim	37	189.14
	Other	52	197.21
	Total	379	
Question 2	Christian	202	189.74
	Hindu	88	190.23
	Muslim	37	185.64
	Other	52	193.71
	Total	379	
Question 3	Christian	202	165.57
	Hindu	88	247.29
	Muslim	37	179.49
	Other	52	195.44
	Total	379	
Question 4	Christian	202	191.25
	Hindu	88	192.85
	Muslim	37	184.76
	Other	52	184.07
	Total	379	
Question 5	Christian	202	194.54
	Hindu	88	188.89
	Muslim	37	179.41
	Other	52	181.77
	Total	379	
Question 6	Christian	202	200.42
	Hindu	88	161.70
	Muslim	37	181.03
	Other	52	203.78
	Total	379	

Table 4.12 Kruskal-Wallis (Ranks):
Religious Groups and Knowledge (continued)

Variables	Religious Groups	N	Mean Rank
Question 7	Christian	202	199.37
	Hindu	88	160.34
	Muslim	37	167.96
	Other	52	219.47
	Total	379	
Question 8	Christian	202	173.70
	Hindu	88	231.52
	Muslim	37	179.61
	Other	52	190.44
	Total	379	
Question 9	Christian	202	166.94
	Hindu	88	244.64
	Muslim	37	173.86
	Other	52	198.59
	Total	379	
Question 10	Christian	202	209.48
	Hindu	88	150.10
	Muslim	37	175.30
	Other	52	192.34
	Total	379	

Source: StatsDirect

Item 1 – students' mean ranks for knowledge of HIV and AIDS: Group C (201.69) more than Group H (159.28), and Group O (197.21) more than Group H (159.28) recognized that HIV and AIDS has an impact on the immune system. With respect to giving the correct response to item 1, Group C obtained the highest mean score.

Item 2 – students' mean ranks for knowledge of HIV: The following paired groups totally dismissed the notion that HIV is spread by casual physical contact: Groups C (165.57) and H (247.29), Groups C (165.57) and O (195.44), Groups H (247.29) and M (179.49), and Groups H (247.29) and O (195.44). Group H carried the highest rank in accepting casual physical contact as a contributing factor to HIV transmission. In comparing Groups C and H and Groups C

**Table 4.13 High School Students
Paired by Religious Groups**

Knowledge Items	High School Students Paired by Religious Groups
AIDS is a disease that weakens the human body's immune system, making it difficult to fight infections and exposing persons infected to a number of serious, often fatal illnesses.	Christian and Hindu; Hindu and Other
HIV is spread from an infected person to a non-infected person through casual physical contact – such as hugging, handshaking, travelling in the same vehicle, touching the same papers, or sharing the same office furniture, telephone or computer.	Christian and Hindu; Christian and Other; Hindu and Muslim; Hindu and Other
If a person tested positive for HIV when he/she takes the antibody test, it does not mean that the person has AIDS. In fact, a person who has AIDS may show no signs or symptoms of the disease and may not develop AIDS for many years.	Christian and Hindu; Other and Hindu
A blood donor cannot get HIV while giving blood.	Christian and Hindu; Other and Hindu
A person can get HIV from animals (such as cats and dogs) around the home and from mosquitoes.	Christian and Hindu; Other and Hindu
A person is likely to contract HIV by being around or working with an infected person on a daily basis and over a long period of time.	Christians and Other; Christian and Hindu; Muslim and Hindu; and Other and Hindu
To protect yourself and/or those you work with from being infected with HIV, you will need to take or put into place preventative measures.	Christian and Hindu

and O, Group C carried the lowest rank, meaning that they were the least likely to accept casual physical contact as a mode of HIV transmission. In contrasting Groups H and M and Groups H and O, we see Group H with the highest mean rank; that is, compared to Groups M and O, Group H was the most likely to see casual physical contact as critical in HIV transmission. Group O followed closely behind Group H with the second highest mean rank.

Item 3 – students' mean ranks for knowledge of HIV and AIDS: The following paired groups indicated that if a person tests positive for HIV, it does not mean that that person has AIDS: Groups C (200.42) and H (161.70) and Groups O (203.78) and H (161.70). When the responses given by Groups C and H were compared, it was noted that Group C persisted in this belief. In comparison to Group H,

Group O did not read negatives in a positive HIV test result. Group O, compared to Groups C and H, demonstrated the highest HIV and AIDS mean score on this item. Group C followed closely behind Group O in mean rank.

Item 4 – students' mean ranks for knowledge of HIV: The following paired groups indicated that a blood donor cannot contract HIV while donating blood: Groups C (199.37) and H (160.34) and Groups O (219.47) and H (160.34). Compared to these two groups (C and H, and O and H), Group O seemed to support the scientific position that there is no hazard at all in donating blood. For this reason, Group O obtained the highest mean score on item 7.

Item 5 – students' mean ranks for knowledge of HIV: The following paired groups indicated that a person can contract HIV from domestic animals: Groups C (173.70) and H (231.52), and Groups O (190.44) and H (231.52). With respect to scores on this item, Group H obtained the highest mean score for incorrect response, followed by Group O, and then Group C.

Item 6 – students' mean ranks for knowledge of HIV: The following paired groups accepted that a person can contract HIV by being with an infected person: Groups C (166.94) and O (198.59), Groups C (166.94) and H (244.64), Groups M (173.86) and H (244.64), and Groups O (198.59) and H (244.64). Groups C and M have the lowest mean scores for incorrect response on this item, while Groups H and O have the highest mean scores for incorrect response.

Item 7 – students' mean ranks for knowledge of HIV: Groups C (209.48) and H (150.10) supported the view that it may be necessary to enact preventive measures against HIV infection. However, Group C has a higher mean for correct score than Group H.

Ethnic Groups

African (81.8%), Indian (52.7%), Chinese (50%), Amerindian (86.7%), Portuguese (40%) and Mixed (37.5%) students showed a moderate knowledge of HIV and AIDS. We tested for any differences in the mean scores for HIV and AIDS knowledge among high school students from different ethnic backgrounds; the hypotheses are:

- $H_0{:}\mu_1 = \mu_2$ There are no differences in the mean scores for HIV and AIDS knowledge among the different ethnicity of high school students. (Null Hypothesis)

- $H_1 : \mu_1 \neq \mu_2$ There are differences in the mean scores for HIV and AIDS knowledge among the different ethnicity of high school students. (Alternative Hypothesis).
- μ_1: refers to similar mean scores for HIV and AIDS knowledge among the different ethnicity of high school students.
- μ_2: refers to different mean scores for HIV and AIDS knowledge among the different ethnicity of high school students.

There are six ethnic groups, so ANOVA may be the appropriate statistical procedure to use. Mention was already made about the assumptions for ANOVA under "Religious Groups". Histograms, normal probability plots and descriptive statistics were used to test these assumptions to ensure that ANOVA is the appropriate procedure to apply.

The histograms and the normal probability plots show a moderate amount of normal distribution of the data, especially as all the normal probability plots approximate a straight line.

Table 4.14 shows that the variances for the ethnic groups are not similar, so the assumption of similarities among variances is not met. The Levene test in table 4.15 also supports this conclusion.

The Levene test of the equality of variance shows that the variances are not equal ($p = 0.000$ is less than $p = 0.05$). Therefore, the K-W test, the nonparametric equivalent of the ANOVA, will be used to compare the median scores for HIV and AIDS knowledge among the various ethnic groups.

The K-W test in table 4.16 shows that there is an overall significant difference ($p = 0.000 < p = 0.05$) in the median scores for HIV and AIDS knowledge among the ethnic groups of high school students. We can, therefore, reject the null hypothesis that there are no differences in HIV and AIDS overall median knowledge scores among the ethnic groups.

Table 4.16 also indicates that students from different ethnic groups showed differences in their median knowledge of HIV and AIDS on six out of ten items; these are 1, 3, 6, 8, 9 and 10 in the following six knowledge areas:

- AIDS is a disease that weakens the human immune system.
- HIV is spread by casual physical contact with infected persons.
- If a person tests positive for HIV, it does not follow that that person has AIDS.
- A person can contract HIV from animals at home or from mosquitoes.
- A person can contract HIV by being with an infected person.
- Protecting oneself as well as co-workers from contracting HIV would necessitate the use of preventive measures

Table 4.16 also indicates that there are significant differences in the median scores for HIV and AIDS knowledge between Africans and Indians (p < 0.0001), between Indians and Amerindians (p = 0.0223), between Mixed and Amerindians (p = 0.0225), and between Africans and Portuguese (p < 0.0001). All the ethnic groups – Indians (52.7%), Africans (81.8%), Amerindians (86.7%), Mixed (37.5%), Portuguese (40%) and Chinese (50%) – showed that they have moderate knowledge of HIV and AIDS. However, African and Amerindian students have relatively better HIV and AIDS knowledge than students from the other ethnic groups.

Figure 4.31 illustrates the statistical significance for the HIV and AIDS knowledge items among the ethnic groups; the significant items are 1, 3, 6, 8, 9 and 10.

The K-W test also identifies students by paired ethnic groups to demonstrate where the differences in median HIV and AIDS knowledge are likely to lie (table 4.18). The K-W test results indicate that there are significant differences in HIV and AIDS knowledge between these pairs (p < 0.05).

Table 4.17 provides the ranking of the mean scores for HIV and AIDS knowledge among the ethnic groups to depict areas of major differences. A high mean rank means a high score and a low mean rank denotes a low score.

Item 1 – students' mean ranks for knowledge of HIV and AIDS: African students (200.81) more than Indian students (182.43) tended to accept the HIV and AIDS has an impact on the immune system. African students have the higher mean score for the correct response to item 1.

Item 3 – students' mean ranks for knowledge of HIV: The following paired groups indicated that HIV is spread by casual physical contact: African (162.69) and Indian (209.62) students, African (162.69) and Mixed (234.01) students, and Mixed (234.01) and Amerindian students (159.00). Mixed students obtained the highest rank, meaning that more than all the ethnic groups, the Mixed group indicated casual physical contact as a contributing factor to HIV transmission. When compared to all the groups, Amerindian students obtained the lowest rank, meaning that they were the least likely to see casual physical contact as a transmission tool. Amerindian students, therefore, obtained the lowest mean score for incorrect response to this item.

Item 6 – students' mean ranks for knowledge of HIV and AIDS: Both African (204.77) and Indian (177.87) students indicated that if a person tests positive for HIV, it does not mean that that person has AIDS. However, when compared to Indian students, African students tended to persist in this belief, and therefore, they obtained the higher mean score for correct response.

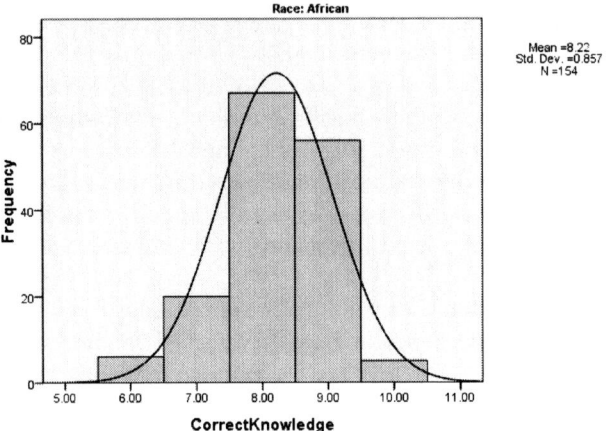

Figure 4.19 Correct knowedge of HIV and AIDS (Africans) – histogram

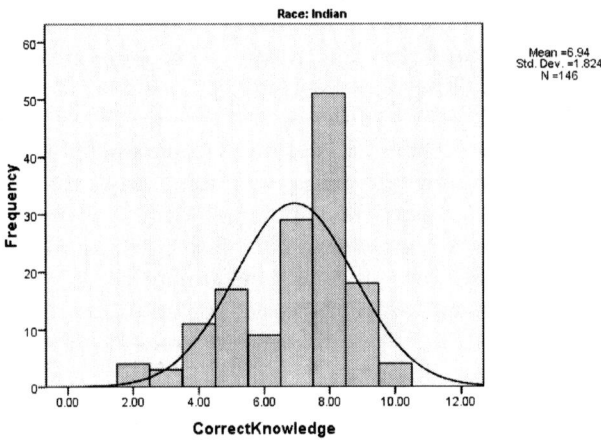

Figure 4.20 Correct knowedge of HIV and AIDS (Indians) – histogram

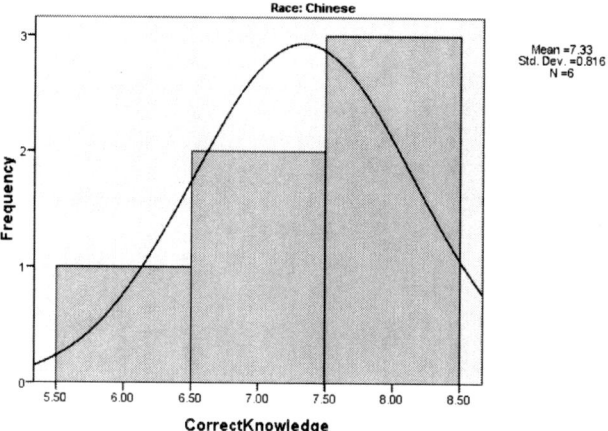

Figure 4.21 Correct knowedge of HIV and AIDS (Chinese) – histogram

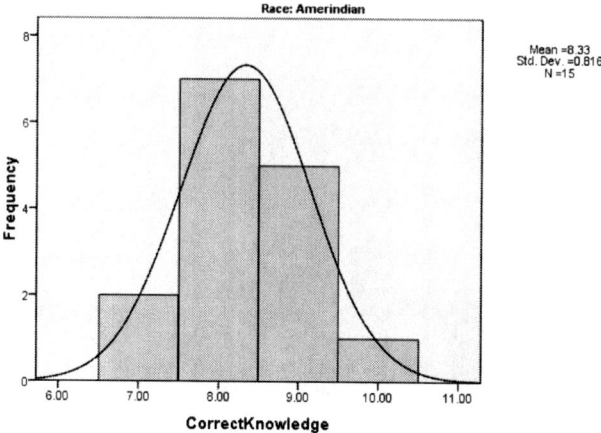

Figure 4.22 Correct knowedge of HIV and AIDS (Amerindians) – histogram

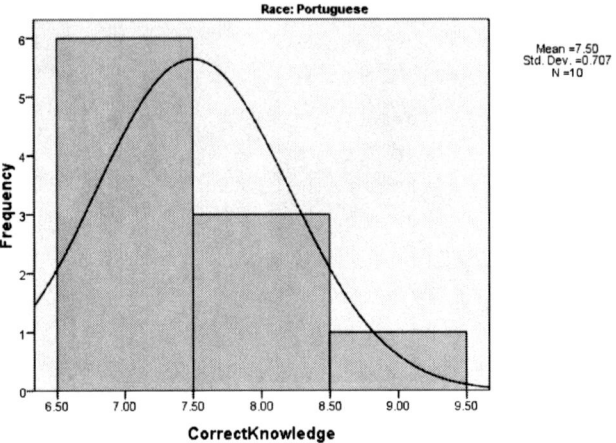

Figure 4.23 Correct knowedge of HIV and AIDS (Portuguese) – histogram

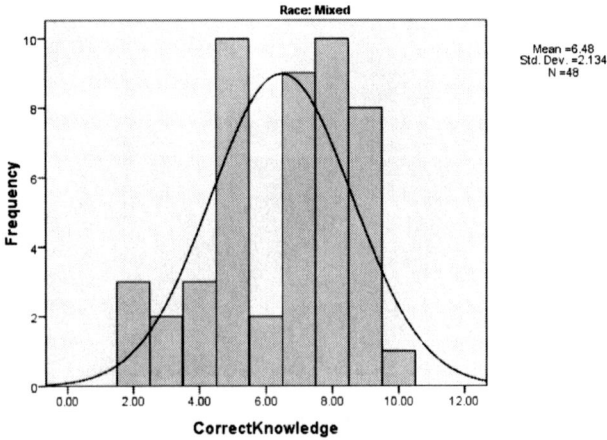

Figure 4.24 Correct knowedge of HIV and AIDS (Mixed) – histogram

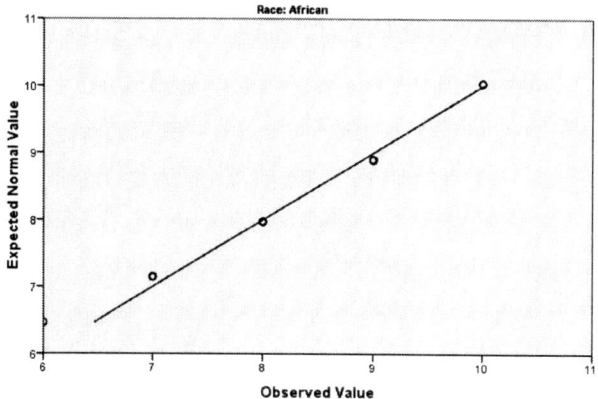

Figure 4.25 Correct knowedge of HIV and AIDS (Africans) – normal
Q-Q plot

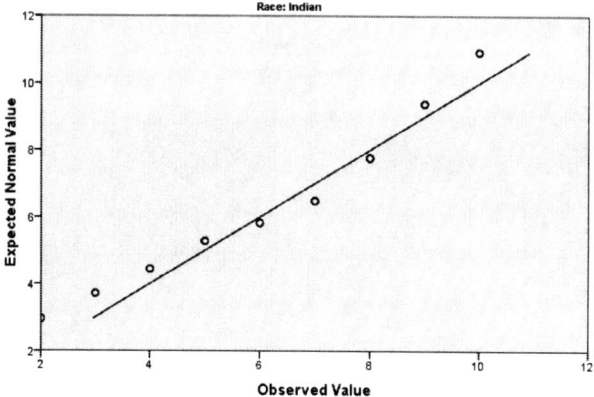

Figure 4.26 Correct knowedge of HIV and AIDS (Indians) – normal
Q-Q plot

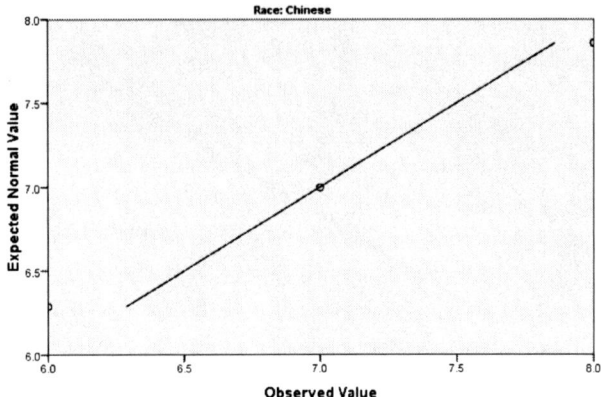

Figure 4.27 Correct knowedge of HIV and AIDS (Chinese) – normal Q-Q plot

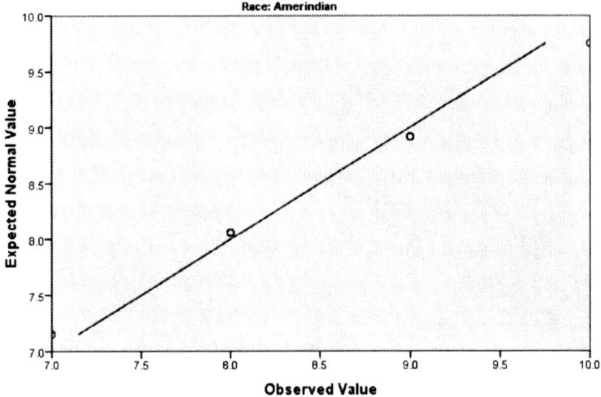

Figure 4.28 Correct knowedge of HIV and AIDS (Amerindians) – normal Q-Q plot

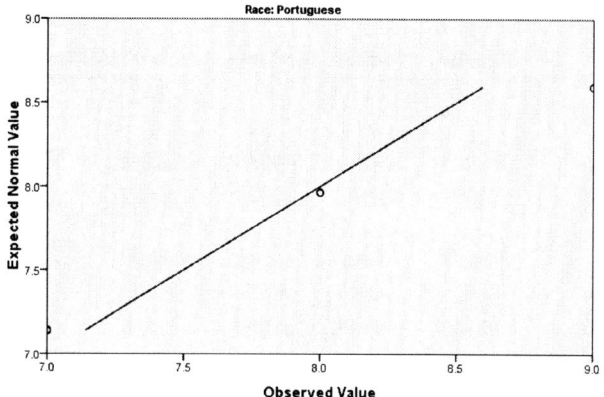

Figure 4.29 Correct knowedge of HIV and AIDS (Portuguese) – normal Q-Q plot

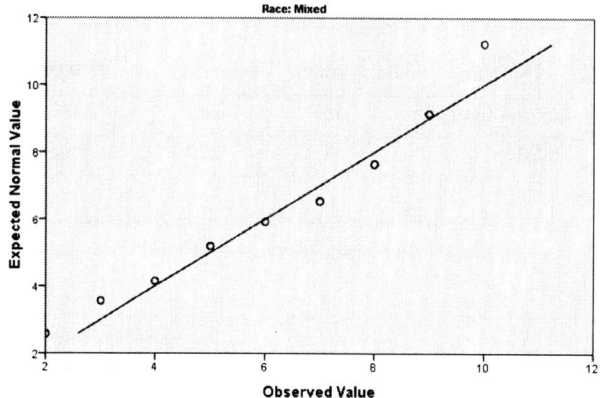

Figure 4.30 Correct knowedge of HIV and AIDS (Mixed) – normal Q-Q plot

Table 4.14 Descriptive Statistics of HIV and AIDS by Ethnic Groups

Descriptive Statistics (Correct Knowledge)	Ethnic Groups					
	African	Indian	Chinese	Amerindian	Portuguese	Mixed
Valid	154	146	6	15	10	48
Missing	0	0	0	0	0	0
Mean	8.2208	6.9384	7.3333	8.3333	7.5000	6.4792
Std. Error of Mean	.06910	.15096	.33333	.21082	.22361	.30798
Median	8.0000	7.5000	7.5000	8.0000	7.0000	7.0000
Mode	8.00	8.00	8.00	8.00	7.00	5.00
Std. Deviation	.85747	1.82406	.81650	.81650	.70711	2.13372
Variance	.735	3.327	.667	.667	.500	4.553
Skewness	−.506	−.855	−.857	.168	1.179	−.512
Std. Error of Skewness	.195	.201	.845	.580	.687	.343
Kurtosis	.225	.124	−.300	−.033	.571	−644
Std. Error of Kurtosis	.389	.399	1.741	1.121	1.334	.674
Range	4.00	8.00	2.00	3.00	2.00	8.00
Minimum	6.00	2.00	6.00	7.00	7.00	2.00
Maximum	10.00	10.00	8.00	10.00	9.00	10.00
Sum	1266.00	1013.00	44.00	125.00	75.00	311.00

Table 4.15 The Levene Test – Ethnic Groups

Levene Statistic	df1	df2	Sig.
20.004	5	373	.000

Table 4.16 Kruskal-Wallis Test Statistics and Pairwise Comparisons – Ethnic Groups

Test Statistics[a, b]

	Correct Knowledge
Chi-Square	64.820
df	5
Asymp. Sig.	.000

a. Kruskal-Wallis Test

b. Grouping Variable: Ethnic Group

Variables	Chi-Square	Df	Asymp. Sig.
Question 1	21.262	5	.001
Question 2	6.700	5	.244
Question 3	58.469	5	.000
Question 4	2.407	5	.790
Question 5	5.866	5	.319
Question 6	17.557	5	.004
Question 7	5.286	5	.382
Question 8	29.973	5	.000
Question 9	55.676	5	.000
Question 10	42.881	5	.000

All Pairwise Comparisons (Dwass-Steel-Chritchlow-Fligner)
Critical q (range) = 4.030092

Group Comparison	Status
Total out of 10~African vs. Total out of 10~Indian	Significant
($|-9.687223| > 4.030092$)	$P < 0.0001$
Total out of 10~Africian vs. Total out of 10~Portuguese	Significant
($|-7.679723| > 4.030092$)	$P < 0.0001$
Total out of 10~Indian vs. Total out of 10~Ethnic Group = 4	Significant
($|4.411995| > 4.030092$)	$P = 0.0223$
Total out of 10~Ethnic Group = 2 vs. Total out of 10~Ethnic Group = 3	Not significant
($|0.192926| > 4.030092$)	$P > 0.9999$
Total out of 10~Ethnic Group = 6 vs. Total out of 10~Ethnic Group = 4	Significant
($|4.408917| > 4.030092$)	$P = 0.0225$

Source: StatsDirect

Item 8 – students' mean ranks for knowledge of HIV: African (170.00) and Indian (204.62) students, and African (170.00) and Mixed (221.11) students believed that a person can contract HIV from domestic animals. Comparisons of the groups' responses revealed that the mixed-race students have the highest mean score for incorrect response, followed by Indian students.

Item 9 – students' mean ranks for knowledge of HIV: The following paired groups indicated that a person can contract HIV by being with an

	Null Hypothesis	Test	Sig.	Decision
1	The distribution of WeakenImmunesystem is the same across categories of Race.	Independent-Samples Kruskal-Wallis Test	.001	Reject the null hypothesis.
2	The distribution of AIDSsymptoms is the same across categories of Race.	Independent-Samples Kruskal-Wallis Test	.244	Retain the null hypothesis.
3	The distribution of Casualphysicalcontact is the same across categories of Race.	Independent-Samples Kruskal-Wallis Test	.000	Reject the null hypothesis.
4	The distribution of Transmisionmethods is the same across categories of Race.	Independent-Samples Kruskal-Wallis Test	.790	Retain the null hypothesis.
5	The distribution of Nontransmissonmethods is the same across categories of Race.	Independent-Samples Kruskal-Wallis Test	.319	Retain the null hypothesis.
6	The distribution of AIDSstatus is the same across categories of Race.	Independent-Samples Kruskal-Wallis Test	.004	Reject the null hypothesis.
7	The distribution of blooddonorisk is the same across categories of Race.	Independent-Samples Kruskal-Wallis Test	.382	Retain the null hypothesis.
8	The distribution of humananimaltransmission is the same across categories of Race.	Independent-Samples Kruskal-Wallis Test	.000	Reject the null hypothesis.
9	The distribution of workingwithHIVpeople is the same across categories of Race.	Independent-Samples Kruskal-Wallis Test	.000	Reject the null hypothesis.
10	The distribution of preventativemeasure is the same across categories of Race.	Independent-Samples Kruskal-Wallis Test	.000	Reject the null hypothesis.

Asymptotic significances are displayed. The significance level is .05.

Figure 4.31 Hypothesis test summary – ethnic groups

infected person: African (163.42) and Indian (209.12) students, African (163.42) and Mixed (233.51) students, and Mixed (233.51) and Amerindian (158.50) students. African and Amerindian students obtained the lowest mean scores for incorrect response to this item, while Indian and mixed-race students obtained the highest mean scores for incorrect response.

Item 10 – students' mean ranks for knowledge of HIV: The following paired groups indicated that it may be necessary to enact preventive measures against HIV infection: African (217.47) and Indian

Table 4.17 Kruskal-Wallis (Ranks):
Ethnic Groups and Knowledge

	Ethnic Group	N	Mean Rank
Weaken Immune System	African	154	200.81
	Indian	146	182.43
	Chinese	6	204.50
	Amerindian	15	204.50
	Portuguese	10	204.50
	Mixed	48	168.97
	Total	379	
AIDS Symptoms	African	154	196.08
	Indian	146	185.42
	Chinese	6	201.00
	Amerindian	15	175.73
	Portuguese	10	182.05
	Mixed	48	189.16
	Total	379	
Casual Physical Contact	African	154	162.69
	Indian	146	209.62
	Chinese	6	190.58
	Amerindian	15	159.00
	Portuguese	10	159.00
	Mixed	48	234.01
	Total	379	
Transmission Methods	African	154	191.31
	Indian	146	187.21
	Chinese	6	195.00
	Amerindian	15	195.00
	Portuguese	10	195.00
	Mixed	48	191.05
	Total	379	
Non-transmission Methods	African	154	191.05
	Indian	146	181.37
	Chinese	6	225.50
	Amerindian	15	212.87
	Portuguese	10	206.55
	Mixed	48	197.86
	Total	379	

Table 4.17 Kruskal-Wallis (Ranks):
Ethnic Groups and Knowledge (continued)

	Ethnic Group	N	Mean Rank
AIDS Status	African	154	204.77
	Indian	146	177.87
	Chinese	6	158.83
	Amerindian	15	222.00
	Portuguese	10	165.15
	Mixed	48	178.57
	Total	379	
Blood Donor Risk	African	154	197.56
	Indian	146	179.18
	Chinese	6	169.67
	Amerindian	15	194.93
	Portuguese	10	163.35
	Mixed	48	205.20
	Total	379	
Human-Animal Transmission	African	154	170.00
	Indian	146	204.62
	Chinese	6	217.17
	Amerindian	15	154.00
	Portuguese	10	172.95
	Mixed	48	221.11
	Total	379	
Working with HIV-infected People	African	154	163.42
	Indian	146	209.12
	Chinese	6	190.08
	Amerindian	15	158.50
	Portuguese	10	158.50
	Mixed	48	233.51
	Total	379	
Preventative Measure	African	154	217.47
	Indian	146	170.42
	Chinese	6	247.00
	Amerindian	15	234.37
	Portuguese	10	171.20
	Mixed	48	144.35
	Total	379	

Table 4.18 High School Students Paired by Ethnicity

Knowledge Items	High School Students Paired by Ethnicity
1. AIDS is a disease that weakens the human body's immune system, making it difficult to fight infections and exposing persons infected to a number of serious, often fatal illnesses.	African and Indian; African and Mixed
2. HIV is spread from an infected person to a non-infected person through casual physical contact – such as hugging, handshaking, travelling in the same vehicle, touching the same papers, or sharing the same office furniture, telephone or computer.	African and Indian; African and Mixed; Mixed and Amerindian
3. If a person tested positive for HIV when he/she takes the antibody test, it does not mean that the person has AIDS. In fact, a person who has AIDS may show no signs or symptoms of the disease and may not develop AIDS for many years.	African and Indian
8. A person can get HIV from animals (such as cats and dogs) around the home and from mosquitoes.	African and Indian; African and Mixed
9. A person is likely to contract HIV by being around or working with an infected person on a daily basis and over a long period of time.	African and Indian; African and Mixed; Mixed and Amerindian
10. To protect yourself and/or those you work with from being infected with HIV, you will need to take or put into place preventative measures.	African and Indian; African and Mixed; Mixed and Amerindian

(170.42) students, African (217.47) and Mixed (144.35) students, and Mixed (144.35) and Amerindian (234.37) students. Amerindian students obtained the highest mean rank for correct response to item 10.

The K-W test results indicated overall that there are statistically significant differences in the median scores for correct HIV and AIDS knowledge ($p < 0.05$) among the ethnic groups. African and Amerindian students had a higher mean rank for correct responses compared to other ethnic groups. How do these groups score on stigma-related attitudes/perceptions?

HIV and AIDS Stigma-related Attitudes/Perceptions

In this study, a sample of high school students in Guyana provided information regarding their attitudes/perceptions of HIV, AIDS and PLHIV. Overall, 60% of the high school students surveyed revealed positive ideas and attitudes toward the virus and the people living with the virus, while 40% portrayed negative ideas and attitudes. The following is an analysis of the attitudes and perceptions revealed by the sampling group.
Negative ideas and attitudes toward HIV, AIDS and PLHIV:

> 94.2% of the students felt that if they were HIV-positive, people would assign them derogatory names and gossip about them;
> 89.7% of the students believed that people make jokes about persons who are HIV-positive;
> 63.6% of the students viewed HIV and AIDS as horrible;
> 59.4% of the students believed that HIV and AIDS is death; and
> 51.2% of the students endorsed the view that HIV and AIDS is punishment.

Students conveyed these negative perceptions/attitudes, notwithstanding their moderate knowledge of HIV and AIDS. The fact that these students scored correctly on an average of about seven out of ten knowledge questions implies that their knowledge of HIV has little impact on their attitudes/perceptions of the virus and persons living with the virus.

Positive ideas and attitudes toward HIV, AIDS and PLHIV:

95.5% of the students thought that anyone could contract HIV, including them;

92.6% of the students did not see HIV and AIDS as a crime;

92.6% of the students held the view that HIV- and AIDS-infected persons should hold employment;

85% of the students indicated that they would be comfortable sharing work tools with an HIV- or AIDS-infected person;

79.7% of the students revealed that they would have no problem shaking hands with an HIV- or AIDS-infected person;

69.1% of the students noted that they would be comfortable sharing the same toilet as an HIV- or AIDS-infected person;

64.9% of the students believed that an HIV- or AIDS-infected person should be able to sell food; and

More than 50% of the students do not believe that a person seen sitting next to an HIV- or AIDS-infected person is also HIV-positive.

The data on HIV and AIDS stigma-related attitudes/perceptions were tested to see if they were normally distributed and to determine the types of statistical procedures to be used for analysing the data.

The histograms, the normal probability plots and the descriptive statistics show that data on HIV and AIDS stigma-related attitudes/perceptions are normally distributed.

In the following table, it is revealed that both male (58.4%) and female (60.6%) high school students scored moderately on positive attitudes/perceptions of HIV, AIDS and PLHIV. Almost two-thirds of Christian and Muslim students have an opposite mindset toward HIV, AIDS and PLHIV; and about two-thirds of African and Amerindian students presented a positive outlook on HIV, AIDS and PLHIV. Both the 13–15 (59.5%) and the 16–18 (59.8%) age groups scored moderately on positive attitudes/perceptions of HIV, AIDS and PLHIV.

The Kendall's W test was used to evaluate respondents' agreement among their rankings of HIV and AIDS stigma-related attitudes/perceptions, and Kendall's W at 0.391 shows that respondents revealed moderate agreement on their rankings. Since the calculated p-value is 0.000, that is, less than $\alpha = 0.05$, then it is appropriate to conclude that Kendall's W is statistically significant, and, therefore, there are significant differences among the rankings for HIV and AIDS stigma-related attitudes/perceptions.

Table 5.1 HIV and AIDS-related Stigma

Variables (Correct Answers)	Frequency		(%)	
	Correct (Appropriate)	Incorrect (Inappropriate)	Correct (Appropriate)	Incorrect (Inappropriate)
HIV and AIDS is death.	154	225	40.6	59.4
HIV and AIDS is punishment.	194	185	48.8	51.2
HIV and AIDS is a crime.	351	28	92.6	7.4
HIV and AIDS can only happen to other people, not me.	362	17	95.5	4.50
HIV and AIDS is horror.	138	241	36.4	63.6
People make jokes about persons who are HIV-positive.	39	340	10.3	89.7
People would assign me names and gossip about me if I were HIV-positive.	22	357	5.8	94.2
People living with HIV or AIDS should be permitted to work.	28	351	7.4	92.6
People living with HIV or AIDS should sell food.	133	246	35.1	64.9
I would be comfortable shaking hands with an HIV- or AIDS-infected person.	77	302	20.3	79.7
I would be comfortable sharing work tools with an HIV- or AIDS-infected person.	57	322	15	85
I would be comfortable sharing the same toilet as an HIV- or AIDS-infected person.	117	262	30.9	69.1
A person seen sitting next to an HIV- or AIDS-infected person is also HIV-positive.	203	176	53.6	46.4
Overall percentage			60	40

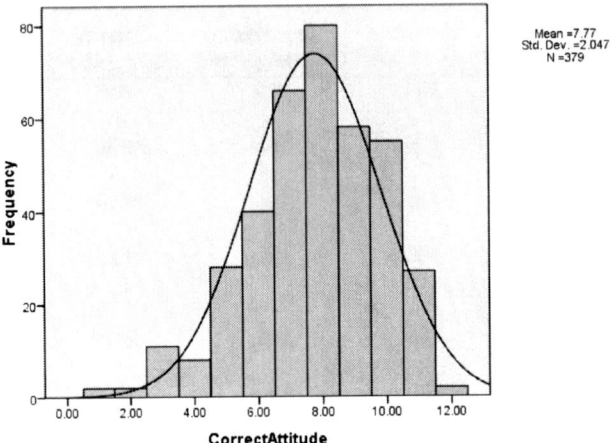

Figure 5.1 HIV and AIDS stigma-related attitudes/perceptions –
histogram

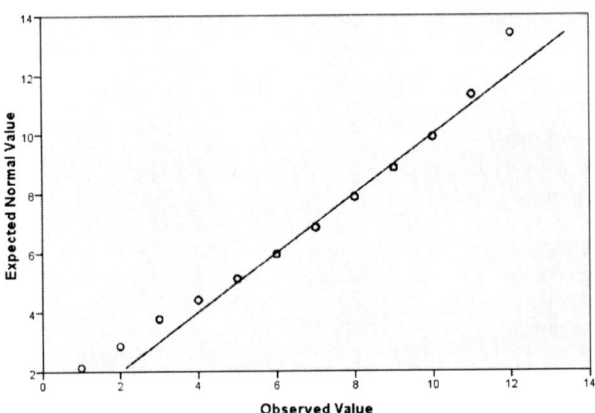

Figure 5.2 HIV and AIDS stigma-related attitudes/perceptions –
normal Q-Q plot

Table 5.2 Descriptive Statistics for Attitudes/Perceptions

Valid	379.000
Missing	.000
Mean	7.773
Std. Error of Mean	.105
Median	8.000
Mode	8.000
Std. Deviation	2.047
Variance	4.192
Skewness	−.530
Std. Error of Skewness	.125
Kurtosis	.171
Std. Error of Kurtosis	.250
Range	11.000
Minimum	1.000
Maximum	12.000
Sum	2946.000

Table 5.3 Demographic Groups vs.
Stigma-related Attitudes/Perceptions

Demographics	Positive Attitudes/ Perceptions n (%)	Negative Attitudes/ Perceptions n (%)	Total n (%)
Gender			
Male	94 (58.4)	67(41.6)	161(42.5)
Female	132(60.6)	86 (39.4)	218 (57.5)
Total	226 (59.6)	153 (40.4)	379
Religious Groups			
Christian	125 (61.9)	77(38.1)	202 (53.3)
Hindu	48 (54.5)	40(45.5)	88 (23.2)
Muslim	23(62.2)	14(37.8)	37 (9.8)
Other	30(57.7)	22(42.2)	52 (13.7)
Total	226 (59.6%)	153 (40.4 %)	379
Ethnic Group/Ethnicity			
African	97 (63)	57(37)	154(40.6)
Indian	85(58.3)	61(41.7)	146(38.5)
Chinese	2(38.3)	4(61.7)	6(1.6)
Amerindian	9(62)	6(38)	16(4)
Portuguese	5(51)	5(49)	10(2.6)
Mixed	28(58.8)	20(41.2)	48(12.7)
Total	226	153	379
Age Group			
Age 13–15	88(59.5)	60 (40.5)	148(39.1)
Age 16–18	137(59.8)	92(40.2)	229(99.5)
Total[a]	226	153	379

a. The 19-and-older age group was removed from the analysis, as there were only two students; for this reason, the total does not add up to 379.

Table 5.4 HIV and AIDS Stigma-related Attitudes/Perceptions

Ranks	
Variables	Mean Rank
Gossip	10.51
Jokes	10.22
Horror	8.52
Death	8.25
Punishment	7.56
Association	7.41
Not selling food	6.67
Not sharing toilet	6.39
Not comfortable	5.71
Not sharing work tools	5.36
Crime	4.87
Not working	4.87
Happens to others	4.68

Table 5.5 Kendall's W Test Statistics

N	379
Kendall's W^a	.391
Chi-Square	1778.575
Df	12

a. Kendall's Coefficient of Concordance

Students ranked the following HIV and AIDS stigma-related attitudes/perceptions as the most important:

1. People would assign me derogatory names and gossip about me if I were HIV-positive.
2. People make jokes about persons who are HIV-positive.
3. HIV and AIDS is horror.
4. HIV and AIDS is death.
5. HIV and AIDS is punishment.
6. A person seen sitting next to an HIV- or AIDS-infected person is also HIV-positive.

Stigma-related Attitudes/Perceptions and Demographics

This section presents the following tests of hypotheses about population means for stigma-related attitudes/perceptions and the demographics of gender, age, religious groups and ethnicity:

- There are no differences in the mean scores for HIV and AIDS stigma-related attitudes/perceptions between male and female high school students.
- There are no differences in the mean scores for HIV and AIDS stigma-related attitudes/perceptions among the different age groups of high school students.
- There are no differences in the mean scores for HIV and AIDS stigma-related attitudes/perceptions among the religious groups.
- There are no differences in the mean scores for HIV and AIDS stigma-related attitudes/perceptions among the ethnic groups.

Gender

To establish if there are any differences in the mean scores for HIV and AIDS stigma-related attitudes/perceptions between male and female high school students, the independent sample t-test was used, since the dependent variable (stigma-related attitudes/perceptions) observations are numeric, and the explanatory variable (male and female students) is dichotomous. The hypotheses for gender are:

- $H_0 : \mu_1 = \mu_2$ There are no differences in the mean scores for HIV and AIDS stigma-related attitudes/perceptions between male and female high school students. (Null Hypothesis).
- $H_1 : \mu_1 \neq \mu_2$ There are differences in the mean scores for HIV and AIDS stigma-related attitudes/perceptions between the male and female high school students. (Alternative Hypothesis)
- μ_1: refers to similar mean levels of HIV and AIDS stigma-related attitudes/perceptions for male and female high school students.
- μ_2: refers to different mean levels of HIV and AIDS stigma-related attitudes/perceptions for male and female high school students.

The t-test assumptions mentioned earlier, the histograms, normal probability plots and descriptive statistics were employed to test these assumptions.

The histograms and normal probability plots on the HIV and AIDS stigma-related attitudes/perceptions of each gender group show that the observations are normally distributed.

The descriptive statistics show a normal distribution between and within gender groups (means and medians are moderately similar between and within gender groups). Since all the t-test assumptions (previously mentioned) have been satisfied, the independent samples t-test was subsequently applied

The comparison of variance shows that there is no need to assume unequal variances. The t-test (table 5.7) provides a t-statistic = −1.396 and a p-value of p = 0.164, which is greater than p = 0.05. Therefore, there is no evidence to reject the null hypothesis. It can be concluded, then, that between the male and female students, there is no significant difference in the mean level of positive attitudes/perceptions of HIV, AIDS and PLHIV. Of those surveyed, 56% of the males and 60.1% of the females showed positive attitudes/perceptions of HIV and AIDS, while 43.5% of the males and 39.9% of the females expressed negative attitudes/perceptions. Overall, there is no statistical significance between the stigma-related attitudes/perceptions shown by both genders, meaning that males and females displayed no differences in the mean scores for HIV and AIDS stigma-related attitudes/perceptions.

The male and female high school students showed no differences in both positive and negative attitudes/perceptions of the virus and people living with the virus.

Those male and female students who provided appropriate responses to attitude/perception items 3, 4, 8, 9, 10, 11 and 12 exhibited positive attitudes/perceptions of HIV, AIDS and PLHIV. Both male and female students did not support the following attitudes/perceptions of HIV, AIDS and PLHIV:

3. HIV and AIDS is a crime.
4. HIV and AIDS only happen to other people, not me.
8. HIV- or AIDS-infected persons should not be permitted to work.
9. HIV- or AIDS-infected persons should not sell food.
10. I would be uncomfortable shaking hands with an HIV- or AIDS-infected person.
11. I would be uncomfortable sharing work tools with an HIV- or AIDS-infected person.
12. I would be uncomfortable sharing the same toilet as an HIV- or AIDS-infected person.

Both male and female students also provided negative responses to items 1, 2, 5, 6, 7 and 13, and, therefore, exhibited inappropriate attitudes/perceptions of HIV, AIDS and PLHIV (table 5.8). These students embraced the following attitudes/perceptions of HIV, AIDS and PLHIV:

1. HIV and AIDS is death.
2. HIV and AIDS is punishment.
5. HIV and AIDS is horror.
6. People make jokes about persons who are HIV-positive.
7. People would assign me names and gossip about me if I were HIV-positive.
13. A person seen sitting next to an HIV- or AIDS-infected person is also HIV-positive.

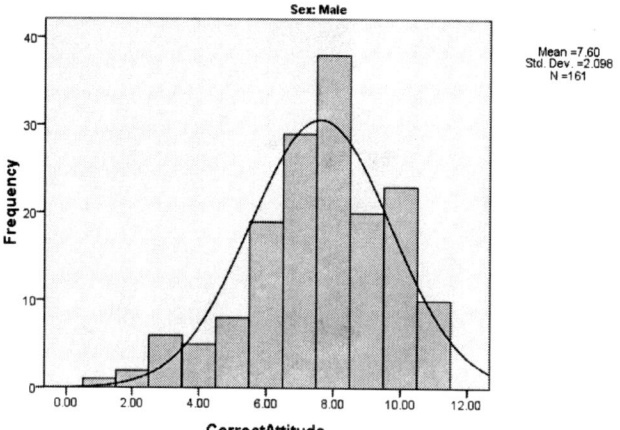

Figure 5.3 Correct attitude/perception of HIV and AIDS (males) – histogram

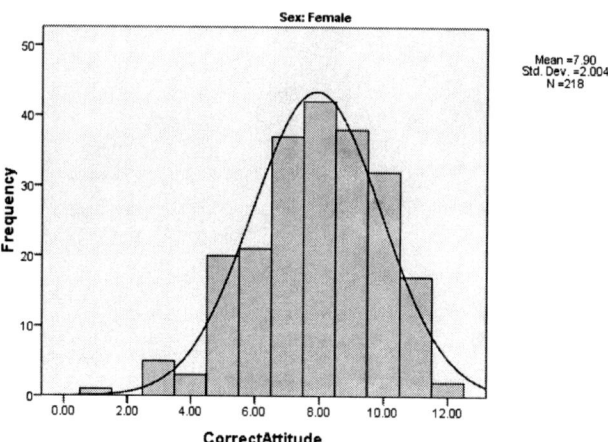

Figure 5.4 Correct attitude/perception of HIV and AIDS (females) – histogram

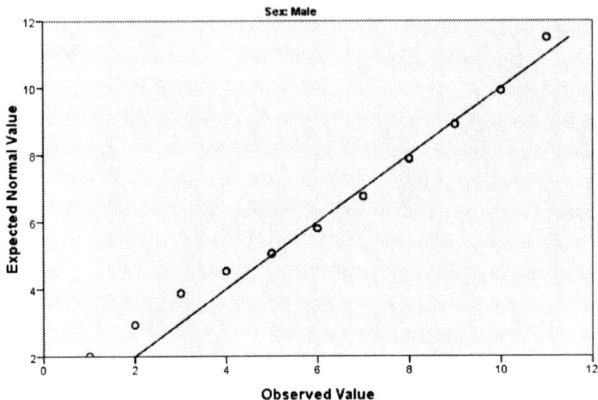

Figure 5.5 Correct attitude/perception of HIV and AIDS (males) – normal Q-Q plot

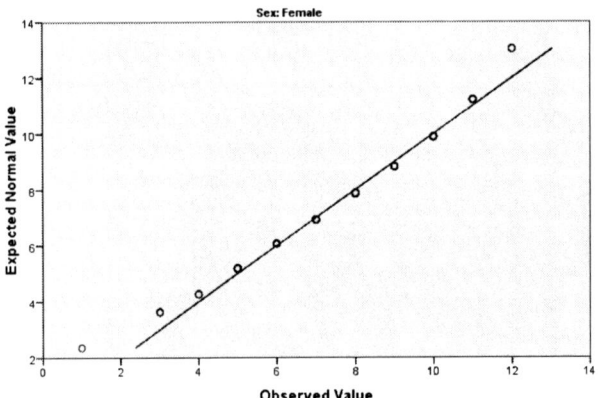

Figure 5.6 Correct attitude/perception of HIV and AIDS (females) – normal Q-Q plot

Table 5.6 Descriptive Statistics by Gender – Male and Female

Descriptive Statistics (Positive Attitudes/Perceptions)	Male	Female
Valid	161.000	218.000
Missing	.000	.000
Mean	7.602	7.899
Std. Error of Mean	.165	.136
Median	8.000	8.000
Mode	8.000	8.000
Std. Deviation	2.098	2.004
Variance	4.403	4.017
Skewness	–.628	–.439
Std. Error of Skewness	.191	.165
Kurtosis	.313	.001
Std. Error of Kurtosis	.380	.328
Minimum	1.000	1.000
Maximum	11.000	12.000

Age

Some 59.5% of the 13–15 age group showed positive attitudes/perceptions of HIV, AIDS and PLHIV, and just under half (40.5%) showed negative attitudes/perceptions. In like manner, just over half (58.1%) of the 16–18 age group showed positive attitudes/perceptions of HIV, AIDS and PLHIV, and just under half (41.9%) showed negative attitudes/perceptions.

To establish whether there are differences in the mean HIV and AIDS stigma-related attitude/perception scores between the 13–15 and 16–18 age groups, the following hypotheses were tested:

- $H_0{:}\mu_1 = \mu_2$ There are no differences in the mean scores for HIV and AIDS stigma-related attitudes/perceptions between the 13–15 and 16–18 age groups of high school students. (Null Hypothesis)
- $H_1{:}\mu_1 \neq \mu_2$ There are differences in the mean scores for HIV and AIDS stigma-related attitudes/perceptions between the 13–15 and 16–18 age groups of high school students. (Alternative Hypothesis)
- μ_1: refers to similar mean levels of HIV and AIDS stigma-related attitudes/perceptions for the 13–15 and 16–18 age groups of high school students.
- μ_2: refers to different mean levels of HIV and AIDS stigma-related attitudes/perceptions for the 13–15 and 16–18 age groups of high school students.

The t-test was used since the dependent variable (stigma-related attitudes/perceptions) observations are numeric, and the explanatory variable (age: 13–15 and 16–18) is dichotomous.

The histograms, normal probability plots and descriptive statistics were employed to test the t-test assumptions.

The histograms with seemingly bell-shaped curves and the normal probability plots approximating a straight line show normal distribution of the observational data on stigma-related attitudes/perceptions.

The descriptive statistics show that the mean, median, variance and range are similar. Therefore, the observational data on stigma-related attitudes/perceptions are normally distributed. The t-test assumptions are satisfied.

The comparison of variance shows that there is no need to assume unequal variances. The t-test (table 5.10) provides a t-statistic = -0.289 and a p-value of $p = 0.773$, which is greater than $p = 0.05$. Therefore, there is no evidence to reject the null hypothesis. It can be concluded, then, that between the 13–15 and 16–18 age groups there is no significant difference in the mean level of positive perceptions/attitudes toward HIV, AIDS and PLHIV.

High school students of the two age groups showed no differences in both positive and negative attitudes/perceptions of HIV, AIDS and PLHIV. Nonetheless, those students in both age groups who provided appropriate responses to attitude/perception items 3, 4, 8, 9, 10, 11 and 12 exhibited positive attitudes/perceptions of HIV, AIDS and PLHIV (table 5.11).

These students did not support the following attitudes/perceptions of HIV, AIDS and PLHIV:

3. HIV and AIDS is a crime.
4. HIV and AIDS only happen to other people, not me.
8. People living with HIV or AIDS should not be permitted to work.
9. People living with HIV or AIDS should not sell food.
10. I would not be comfortable shaking hands with an HIV- or AIDS-infected person.
11. I would not be comfortable sharing work tools with an HIV- or AIDS-infected person.
12. I would not be comfortable sharing the same toilet as an HIV- or AIDS-infected person.

Both age groups also provided negative responses to items 1, 2, 5, 6, 7 and 13, and, therefore, exhibited inappropriate attitudes/perceptions of HIV, AIDS and PLHIV (table 5.11).

Table 5.7 Unpaired t-test for Gender and Attitudes/Perceptions

Independent Samples Test

		Levene's Test for Equality of Variances		t-test for Equality of Means						95% Confidence Interval of the Difference	
		F	Sig.	t	Df	Sig. (2-tailed)	Mean Difference	Std. Error Difference		Lower	Upper
Correct Attitude	Equal variances assumed	.113	.737	−1.396	377	.164	−.29660	.21249		−.71441	.12121
	Equal variances not assumed			−1.386	335.833	.167	−.29660	.21396		−71747	.12428

Source: StatsDirect

Table 5.8 HIV and AIDS Stigma-related Attitudes and Perceptions

Variables/Question	Appropriate n (%)			Inappropriate n (%)		
	Male n (%)	Female n (%)	Total N (%)	Male n (%)	Female n (%)	Total N (%)
Question 1	69 (42.9)	85 (39)	154 (40.6)	92 (57.1)	133 (61)	225 (59.4)
Question 2	77 (47.8)	117 (53.7)	194 (51.2)	84 (52.2)	101 (46.3)	185 (48.8)
Question 3	145 (90.1)	206 (94.5)	351 (92.6)	16 (9.9)	12 (5.5)	28 (7.4)
Question 4	152 (94.4)	210 (96.3)	362	9 (5.6)	8 (3.9)	17
Question 5	57 (35.4)	81 (37.2)	138 (36.4)	104 (64.6)	137 (62.8)	241 (63.6)
Question 6	15 (9.3)	24 (11)	39 (10.3)	146 (90.7)	194 (89)	340 (89.7)
Question 7	11 (3.1)	11 (5)	22 (5.8)	150 (96.9)	207 (95)	357 (94.2)
Question 8	152 (94.4)	199 (91.3)	351 (92.6)	9 (5.6)	19 (8.7)	28 (7.4)
Question 9	98 (60.9)	148 (67.9)	246 (64.9)	63 (39.1)	70 (32.1)	133 (35.1)
Question 10	120 (74.5)	182 (83.5)	302 (79.7)	41 (25.5)	36 (16.5)	77 (20.3)
Question 11	133 (82.6)	189 (86.7)	322 (84.7)	28 (17.4)	29 (13.3)	57 (15.3)
Question 12	111 (68.9)	151 (69.3)	262 (69.1)	50 (31.1)	67 (30.7)	117 (30.9)
Question 13	84 (52.2)	119 (54.6)	203 (53.6)	77 (47.8)	99 (45.4)	176 (46.4)

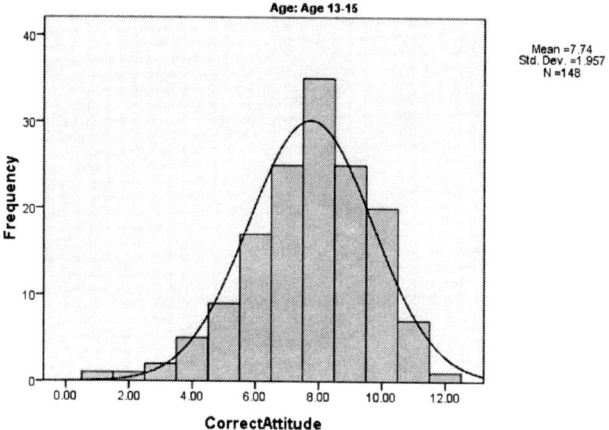

Figure 5.7 Correct attitude/perception of HIV and AIDS (13–15 yrs) – histogram

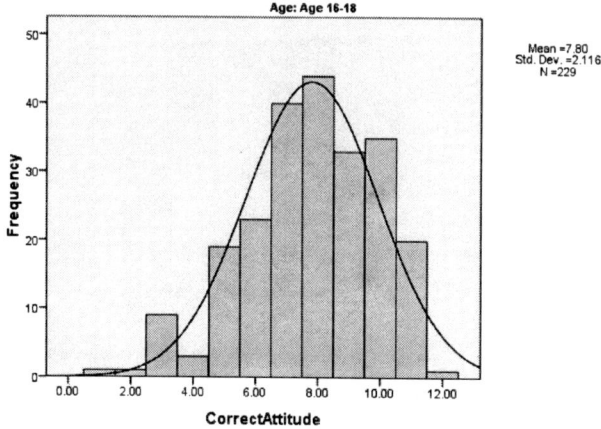

Figure 5.8 Correct attitude/perception of HIV and AIDS (16–18 yrs) – histogram

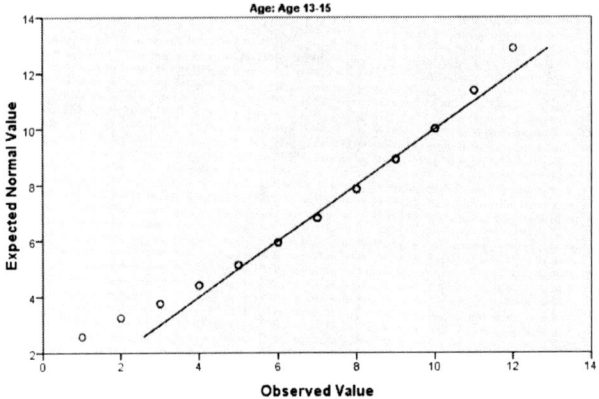

Figure 5.9 Correct attitude/perception of HIV and AIDS (13–15 yrs) – normal Q-Q plot

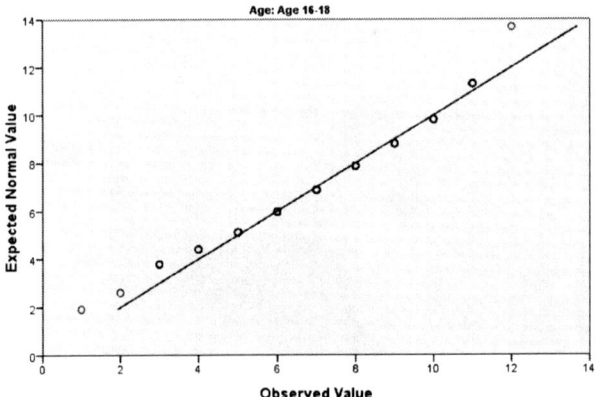

Figure 5.10 Correct attitude/perception of HIV and AIDS (16–18 yrs) – normal Q-Q plot

Table 5.9 Descriptive Statistics for Positive Attitudes/ Perceptions by Age Groups

Descriptive Statistics (Positive Attitudes/Perceptions)	13–15 yrs	16–18yrs
Valid	148.00	229.00
Missing	.00	.00
Mean	7.74	7.80
Std. Error of Mean	.16	.14
Median	8.00	8.00
Mode	8.00	8.00
Std. Deviation	1.96	2.12
Variance	3.83	4.48
Skewness	–60	–50
Std. Error of Skewness	.20	.16
Kurtosis	.57	–03
Std. Error of Kurtosis	.40	.32
Range	11.00	11.00
Minimum	1.00	1.00
Maximum	12.00	12.00
Sum	1145.00	1786.00

Both age groups showed the following attitudes/perceptions toward PLHIV:

1. HIV and AIDS is death.
2. HIV and AIDS is punishment.
5. HIV and AIDS is horror.
6. People make jokes about persons who are HIV-positive.
7. People would assign me names and gossip about me if I were HIV-positive.
13. A person seen sitting next to an HIV- or AIDS-infected person is also HIV-positive.

Religious Groups

Christian (63.4%), Hindu (43.2%), Muslim (64.9%) and Other (61.5%) high school students scored moderately on positive attitudes/perceptions of HIV, AIDS and PLHIV. Even so, one needs to determine if there are differences in the mean score for HIV and AIDS stigma-related attitudes/perceptions of high school students from different religious persuasions. To make this determination, one has to test the following:

- $H_0: \mu_1 = \mu_2$ There are no differences in the mean scores for HIV and AIDS stigma-related attitudes/perceptions among the different religious persuasions. (Null Hypothesis).

- $H_1 : \mu_1 \neq \mu_2$ There are differences in the mean scores for HIV and AIDS stigma-related attitudes/perceptions among the different religious persuasions. (Alternative Hypothesis)
- μ_1: refers to similar mean HIV and AIDS stigma-related attitude/perception scores of high school students from different religious persuasions.
- μ_2: refers to different mean HIV and AIDS stigma-related attitude/perception scores of high school students from different religious persuasions.

In view of the fact that there are more than two groups (Christians, Hindus, Muslims and Others), the t-test is not appropriate. Therefore, the ANOVA was used. The assumptions of ANOVA were mentioned earlier.

The histograms, the normal probability plots and descriptive statistics were applied to test the ANOVA assumptions.

The histograms and the normal probability plots show a normal distribution of the data on the positive perceptions/attitudes of religious groups toward HIV, AIDS and PLHIV.

The descriptive statistics show that the variances are not similar, but the data are normally distributed vis-à-vis the similarity of means, medians and ranges.

Assumptions 3 and 4 of ANOVA are satisfied. The Levene F test has a p-value of 0.109, and since it is greater than $p = 0.05$, there is no evidence to reject the null hypothesis of no differences in variances. The variances, therefore, are similar. Thus, the assumption that the variances have to be similar is satisfied. The test showing equality of variance indicates that it should be assumed that there is equal variance in stigma-related attitudes/perceptions among the religious groups. Therefore, the ANOVA procedure was used (see appendix 3).

With $F = 5.404$ and $p = 0.001$, which is less than the p-value of 0.05, it can be concluded that there are differences in the mean HIV and AIDS stigma-related attitudes/perceptions among the religious groups. Hence, there is a relationship between religious beliefs and stigma-related attitudes/perceptions. There is also statistical significance ($p < 0.05$) for the mean HIV and AIDS stigma-related attitudes/perceptions in three areas among the four religious groups of high school students. These results imply that students' religious persuasions affect their attitudes/perceptions of HIV, AIDS and PLHIV, indicating that the mean scores for the four religious groups are not equal in the following three areas of HIV and AIDS stigma-related attitudes/perceptions:

- HIV and AIDS is a crime.
- I would not be comfortable sharing work tools with an HIV- or AIDS-infected person.
- I would not be comfortable sharing the same toilet as an HIV- or AIDS-infected person.

Table 5.10 Unpaired t-test for Age Groups and Attitudes/Perceptions

Independent Samples Test

		Levene's Test for Equality of Variances		t-test for Equality of Means					95% Confidence Interval of the Difference	
		F	Sig.	t	df	Sig. (2-tailed)	Mean Difference	Std. Error Difference	Lower	Upper
Correct Attitude	Equal variances assumed	1.526	.218	-.289	375	.773	-.06264	.21673	-.48879	.36351
	Equal variances not assumed			-.294	331.205	.769	-.06264	.21311	-.48186	.35658

Source: StatsDirect

Table 5.11 Stigma-related Attitudes and Perceptions by Age Groups

Statements	Appropriate (n %)				Inappropriate (n %)		
	13–15 yrs N=148 n (%)	16–18yrs N =229 n (%)	19 and over N = 2 n (%)	Total N (%)	13–15 n (%)	16–18 n (%)	Total N (%)
Question 1	60 (40.5)	94 (69.6)	0 (0)	154 (40.6)	88 (59.5)	135 (30.4)	225 (59.4)
Question 2	74 (50)	119 (52)	1 (50)	194 (51.2)	74 (50)	110 (48)	185 (48.8)
Question 3	134 (90.5)	215 (93.9)	2 (100)	351 (92.6)	14 (9.5)	14 (6.1)	28 (7.4)
Question 4	144 (97.3)	216 (94.3)	2 (100)	362 (95.5)	4 (2.7)	13 (5.7)	17 (4.5)
Question 5	47 (31.8)	90 (39.3)	1 (50)	138 (36.4)	101 (68.2)	139 (60.7)	241 (63.6)
Question 6	15 (10.1)	24 (10.5)	0 (0)	39 (10.3)	133 (89.9)	205 (89.5)	340 (89.7)
Question 7	10 (6.8)	12 (5.2)	0 (0)	22 (5.8)	138 (93.2)	217 (94.8)	357 (94.2)
Question 8	138 (93.2)	211 (92.1)	2 (100)	351 (93.2)	10 (6.8)	18 (7.9)	28 (6.8)
Question 9	100 (67.6)	145 (63.3)	1 (50)	246 (64.9)	48 (32.4)	84 (36.7)	133 (35.1)
Question 10	123 (83.1)	178 (77.7)	1 (50)	302 (79.7)	25 (16.9)	51 (22.3)	77 (20.3)
Question 11	127 (85.8)	193 (84.3)	2 (100)	322 (85)	21 (14.2)	36 (15.7)	57 (15)
Question 12	100 (67.6)	160 (69.7)	2 (100)	262 (69.1)	48 (32.4)	69 (30.3)	117 (30.9)
Question 13	73 (49.3)	129 (56.3)	1 (50)	203 (53.7)	75 (50.7)	100 (43.7)	176 (46.3)

A = Appropriate attitude
NA = Not Appropriate Attitude

These responses – HIV and AIDS is a crime [F (3,375) = 3.70, p < 0.05]; I would not be comfortable sharing work tools with an HIV- or AIDS-infected person [F (3,375) = 3.487, p < 0.05]; and I would not be comfortable sharing the same toilet as an HIV- or AIDS-infected person [F (3,375) = 5.356, p < 0.05] – differ among the four religious groups of high school students. These test results, however, do not show which of the four religious groups differ from one another; therefore, the Games-Howell test was used to make this determination. The Games-Howell test was chosen because it does not assume equal variances and group sizes, and the results show unequal variances and group sizes for the four religious groups. The Tukey test was not applied because it is parametric and assumes equal variances and equal group sizes.

The Games-Howell test (appendix 4) identified two other stigma-related attitudes/perceptions:

1. The perception that "HIV and AIDS is death" is significant between the Christian and Hindu students.
2. The perception that "HIV and AIDS only happen to other people, not me" is significant between the Christian and Muslim students.

Table 5.9 shows these two stigma-related attitudes/perceptions plus the three others found earlier to be statistically significant.

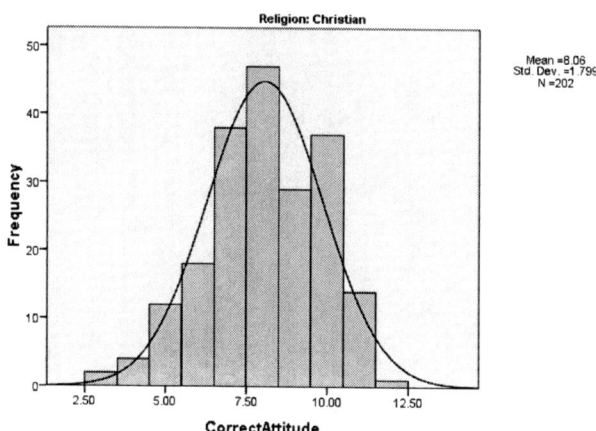

Figure 5.11 Correct attitude/perception of HIV and AIDS (Christians) – histogram

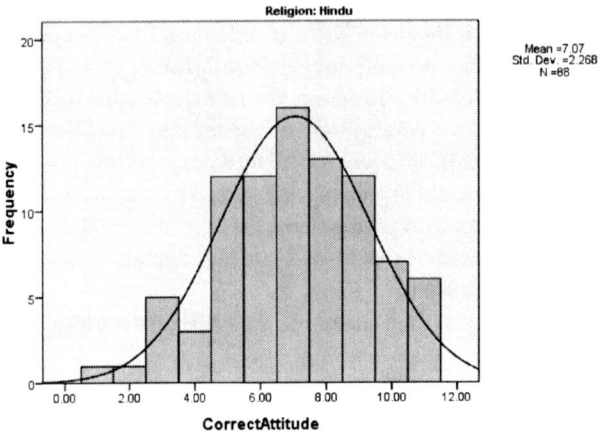

Figure 5.12 Correct attitude/perception of HIV and AIDS (Hindus) – histogram

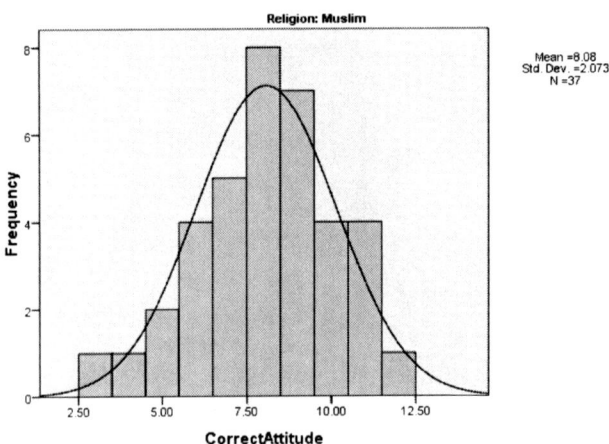

Figure 5.13 Correct attitude/perception of HIV and AIDS (Muslims) – histogram

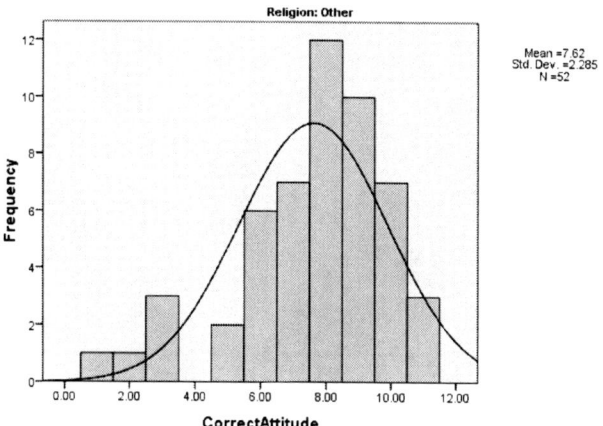

Figure 5.14 Correct attitude/perception of HIV and AIDS (others) – histogram

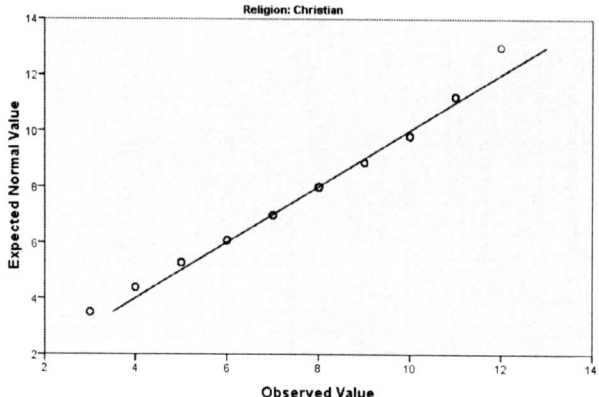

Figure 5.15 Correct attitude/perception of HIV and AIDS (Christians) – normal Q-Q plot

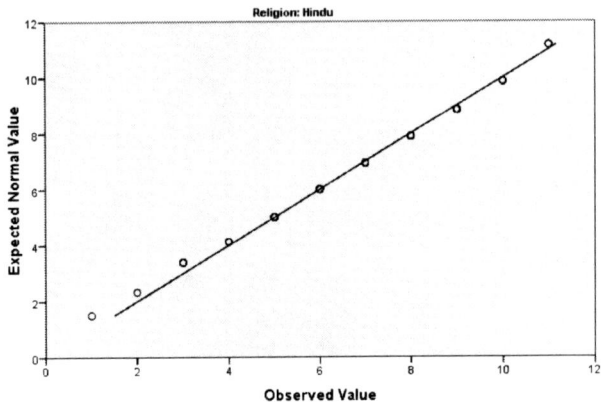

Figure 5.16 Correct attitude/perception of HIV and AIDS (Hindus) – normal Q-Q plot

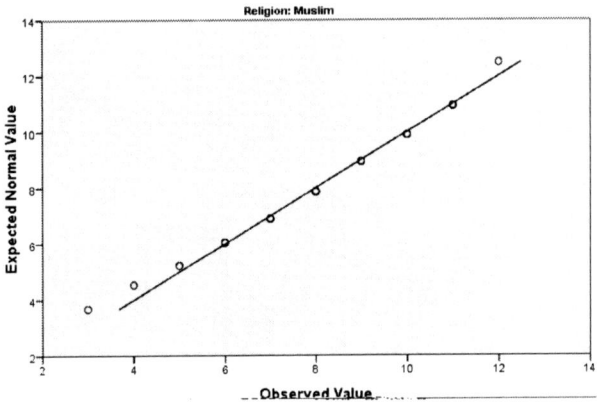

Figure 5.17 Correct attitude/perception of HIV and AIDS (Muslims) – normal Q-Q plot

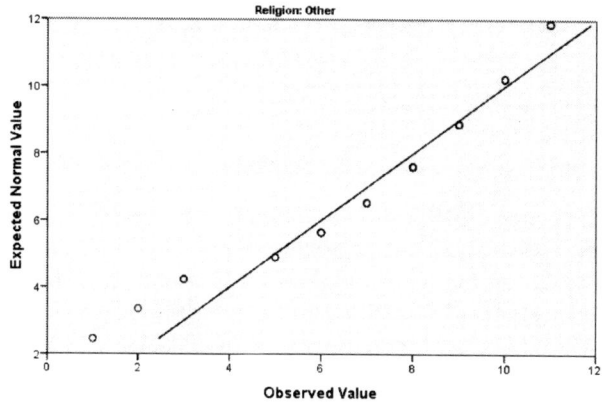

Figure 5.18 Correct attitude/perception of HIV and AIDS (others) –
normal Q-Q plot

**Table 5.12 Descriptive Statistics by Religious Groups
and Attitudes/Perceptions**

Descriptive Statistics (Positive Attitudes/ Perceptions)	Christian	Hindu	Muslim	Other
Valid	202.000	88.000	37.000	52.000
Missing	.000	.000	.000	.000
Mean	8.064	7.068	8.081	7.615
Std. Error of Mean	.127	.242	.341	.317
Median	8.000	7.000	8.000	8.000
Mode	8.000	7.000	8.000	8.000
Std. Deviation	1.799	2.268	2.073	2.285
Variance	3.235	5.145	4.299	5.222
Skewness	−.320	−262	−.351	−1.001
Std. Error of Skewness	.171	.257	.388	.330
Kurtosis	−271	−.308	−.086	.911
Std. Error of Kurtosis	.341	.508	.759	.650
Range	9.000	10.000	9.000	10.000
Minimum	3.000	1.000	3.000	1.000
Sum	1629.000	622.000	299.000	396.000

Table 5.13 The Levene F Test and Attitudes/Perceptions – Religious Groups

Approximate Equality of Variance Tests
Levene's (W50) F = 2.030923 (df = 3,375) P = 0.1091
Bartlett's chi-square = 9.217689 df = 3 P = 0.0265

Source: StatsDirect

The Games-Howell test shows the following results:

Item 1 – (HIV and AIDS is death.): The Christian high school students' mean attitude/perception score for item 1 significantly differs from that of the Hindu high school students (p < 0.05). The Christian students obtained a significantly higher mean score for positive attitudes/perceptions of HIV, AIDS and PLHIV than the Hindu students, in that Christian more than Hindu students did not view HIV and AIDS as death.

Item 2 – (HIV and AIDS is a crime.): The Christian high school students' mean attitude/perception score for item 2 significantly differs from that of the Hindu high school students (p < 0.05). The Christian students obtained a significantly higher mean score for positive attitudes/perceptions of HIV, AIDS and PLHIV than the Hindu students, in that Christian more than Hindu students would more than likely not perceive HIV and AIDS as a crime.

Item 3 – (HIV happens to other people, not me.): The Christian high school students' mean attitude/perception score for item 3 significantly differs from that of the Muslim high school students (p < 0.05). The Muslim students obtained a significantly higher mean score for positive attitudes/perceptions of HIV, AIDS and PLHIV than the Christian students, in that Muslim more than Christian students would not subscribe to the view that "HIV and AIDS only happen to other people, not me".

Table 5.14 High School Students Paired by Religious Groups

Stigma-related Attitudes/Perceptions Items	High School Students Paired by Religious Groups
1. HIV and AIDS is death.	Christian and Hindu
2. HIV and AIDS is a crime.	Christian and Hindu
3. HIV happens to other people, not me.	Christian and Muslim

Table 5.14 High School Students Paired
by Religious Groups (continued)

Stigma-related Attitudes/Perceptions Items	High School Students Paired by Religious Groups
4. I would not be comfortable sharing work tools with an HIV- or AIDS-infected person.	Christian and Hindu
5. I would not be comfortable sharing the same toilet as an HIV- or AIDS-infected person.	Christian and Hindu; Hindu and Other

Item 4 – (I would not be comfortable sharing work tools with an HIV- or AIDS-infected person.): The Christian students' mean attitude/perception score for item 4 significantly differs from that of the Hindu students ($p < 0.05$). The Christian students received a significantly higher mean score for positive attitude/perception of HIV, AIDS and PLHIV than the Hindu students, in that Christian more than Hindu students would feel comfortable sharing work tools with an HIV- or AIDS-infected person.

Item 5 – (I would not be comfortable sharing the same toilet as an HIV- or AIDS-infected person.): The Christian students' mean attitude/perception score for item 5 significantly differs from that of the Hindu students ($p < 0.05$). The Christian students received a higher mean score for positive attitudes/perceptions of HIV, AIDS and PLHIV than the Hindu students, in that Christian more than Hindu students would feel comfortable sharing a toilet with an HIV- or AIDS-infected person. Additionally, the Hindu students' mean attitude/perception score for item 5 significantly differs from students of Other religious affiliations ($p < 0.05$). The Hindu students obtained a higher mean score for positive attitudes/perceptions of HIV, AIDS and PLHIV than the students of Other religious groups, in that Hindu more than Other students would feel comfortable sharing a toilet with an HIV- or AIDS-infected person.

Ethnic Groups

African (66.9%), Indian (52.7%), Chinese (33.3%), Amerindian (60%), Portuguese (30%) and Mixed (58.3%) showed moderate scores on positive attitudes/perceptions toward HIV, AIDS and PLHIV.

Since there are six ethnic groups, the ANOVA was applied to test the null hypothesis that the means of all these groups are equal.

- $H_0 : \mu_1 = \mu_2$ There are no differences in the mean scores for HIV and AIDS stigma-related attitudes/perceptions among the different ethnic groups of high school students. (Null Hypothesis)
- $H_1 : \mu_1 \neq \mu_2$ There are differences in the mean scores for HIV and AIDS stigma-related attitudes/perceptions among the different ethnic groups of high school students. (Alternative Hypothesis)
- μ_1: refers to similar mean HIV and AIDS stigma-related attitudes/perceptions for different ethnicities.
- μ_2: refers to different mean HIV and AIDS stigma-related attitudes/perceptions for different ethnicities.

But first, prior to applying the ANOVA procedure, the assumptions of the ANOVA (already indicated in this text) have to be tested to ensure that its assumptions are satisfied. The histograms, the normal probability plots and descriptive statistics were used to test these assumptions.

The histograms and the normal probability plots suggest that the data on ethnicity and stigma-related attitudes/perceptions may not be normally distributed. In addition, the descriptive statistics indicate that the means and medians are not equal.

The test of the equality of variance shows that the variances also are not equal ($p = 0.021$ is less than $p = 0.05$). Therefore, the Kruskal-Wallis (K-W) test, the non-parametric equivalent of the ANOVA, was used to compare the median for positive HIV and AIDS attitudes/perceptions of the ethnic groups.

Table 5.17 shows that the K-W test indicates that there is an overall significant difference ($p = 0.011 < 0.05$) in the median score for positive HIV and AIDS attitudes/perceptions among the ethnic groups of high school students. We can, therefore, reject the null hypothesis that there are no differences in overall median attitudes/perceptions scores among the ethnic groups. Table 5.18 also indicates statistical significance in three areas of attitudes/perceptions: HIV and AIDS is death ($p = 0.025 < p = 0.05$); not sharing work tools ($p = 0.004 < p = 0.05$); and not sharing toilet ($p = .004 < p = 0.05$).

Appendix 5 shows the mean ranks of the attitudes/perceptions of the different ethnic groups. A high mean rank denotes a high score and a low mean rank denotes a low score.

Item 1: African (172.25) more than Mixed (219.63) students are less likely to see HIV and AIDS as death. African students obtained the lower mean score for negative attitudes/perceptions of HIV, AIDS and PLHIV.

Item 2: African (179.96) more than Chinese (287.83) students are less likely to be uncomfortable with sharing work tools with an HIV- or AIDS-infected person; and Indian (193.95) compared to Chinese (287.83) students are less likely to be uncomfortable. Chinese students obtained the highest mean score for negative attitudes/ perceptions of HIV, AIDS and PLHIV.

Item 3: African (177.03) more than Chinese (289.42) students are less likely to be uncomfortable with sharing a toilet with an HIV- or AIDS-infected person; Amerindian (156.77) more than Chinese (289.42) students are less likely to be uncomfortable. Chinese students obtained the highest mean score for negative attitudes/ perceptions of HIV, AIDS and PLHIV.

The K-W test results indicated that there are statistically significant differences in median scores for only three out of thirteen stigma-related attitudes/perceptions among the ethnic groups. However, does good knowledge of HIV and AIDS produce positive attitudes/perceptions? Prior to answering this question, determining the predictive capacity of age, religion and ethnicity, which are hypothesized in this study as predictors of HIV and AIDS knowledge, is required.

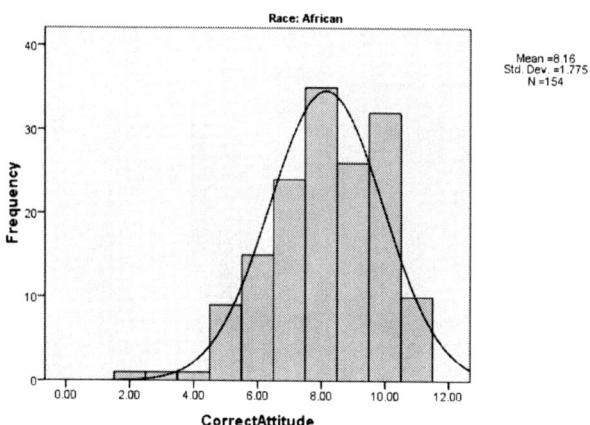

Figure 5.19 Correct attitude/perception of HIV and AIDS (Africans) – histogram

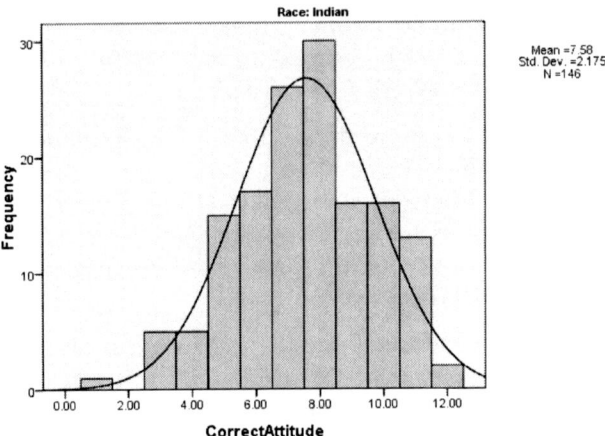

Figure 5.20 Correct attitude/perception of HIV and AIDS (Indians) – histogram

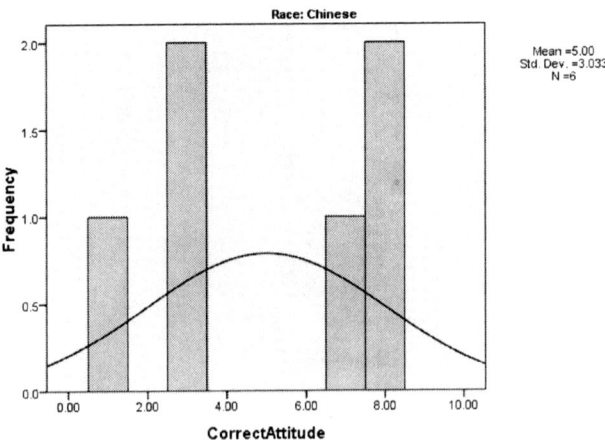

Figure 5.21 Correct attitude/perception of HIV and AIDS (Chinese) – histogram

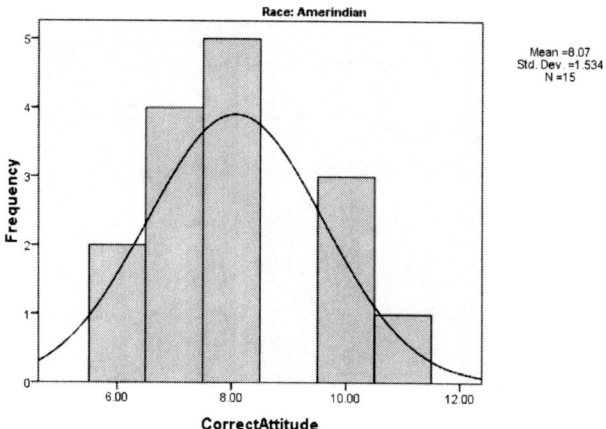

Figure 5.22 Correct attitude/perception of HIV and AIDS (Amerindians) – histogram

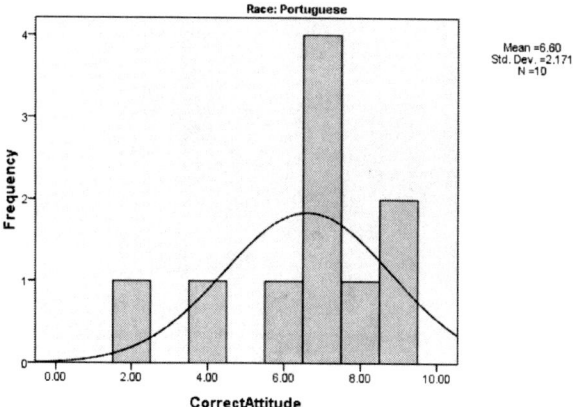

Figure 5.23 Correct attitude/perception of HIV and AIDS (Portuguese) – histogram

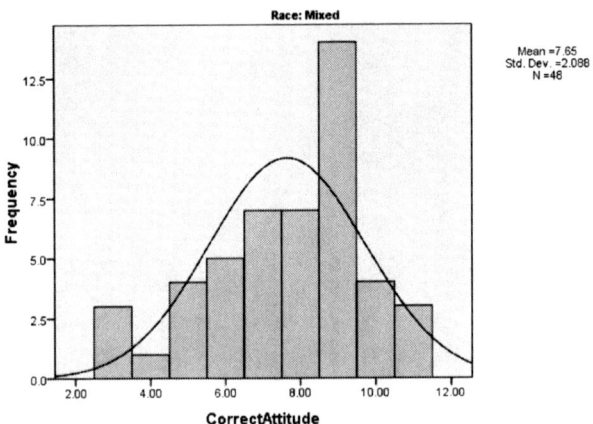

Figure 5.24 Correct attitude/perception of HIV and AIDS (Mixed) – histogram

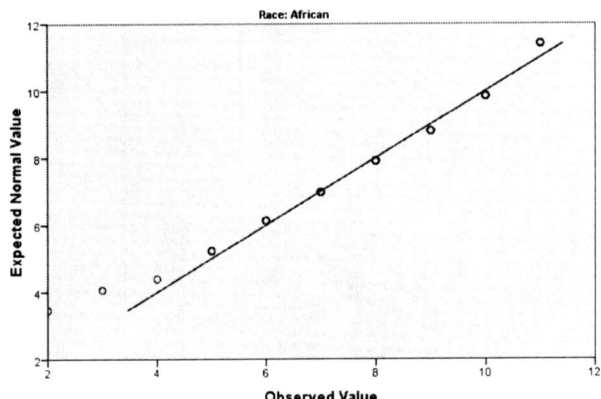

Figure 5.25 Correct attitude/perception of HIV and AIDS (Africans) – normal Q-Q plot

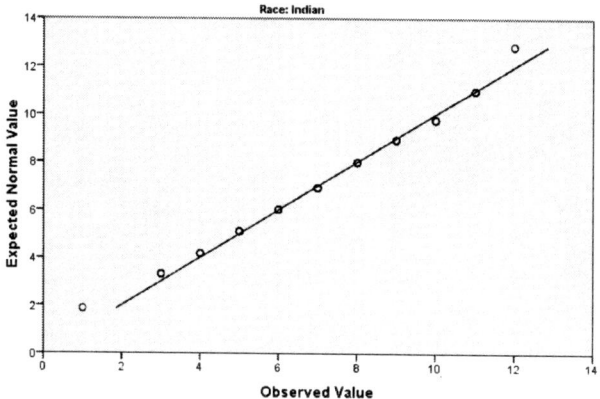

Figure 5.26 Correct attitude/perception of HIV and AIDS (Indians) – normal Q-Q plot

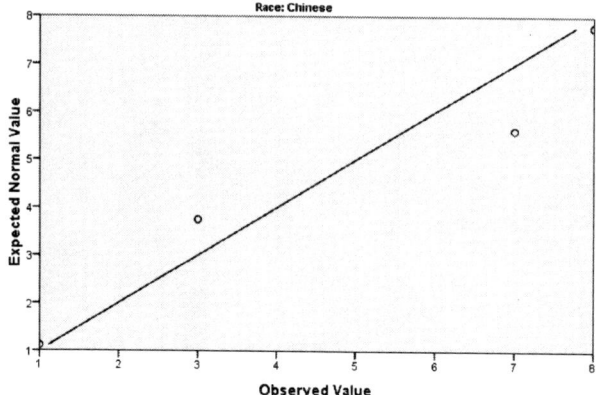

Figure 5.27 Correct attitude/perception of HIV and AIDS (Chinese) – normal Q-Q plot

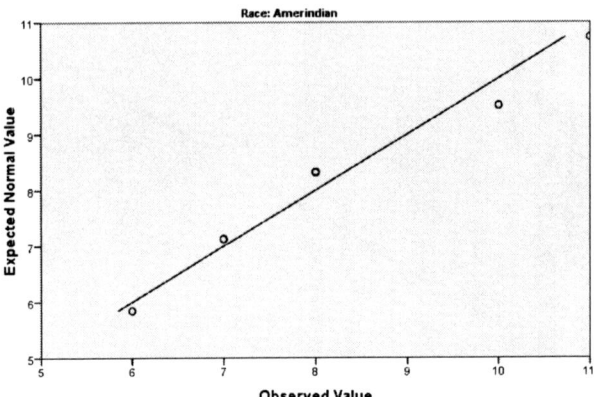

Figure 5.28 Correct attitude/perception of HIV and AIDS
(Amerindians) – normal Q-Q plot

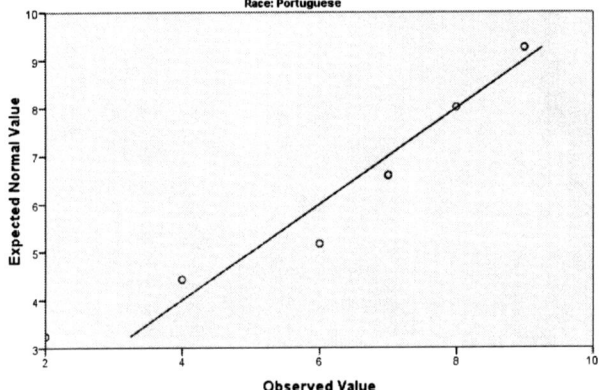

Figure 5.29 Correct attitude/perception of HIV and AIDS
(Portuguese) – normal Q-Q plot

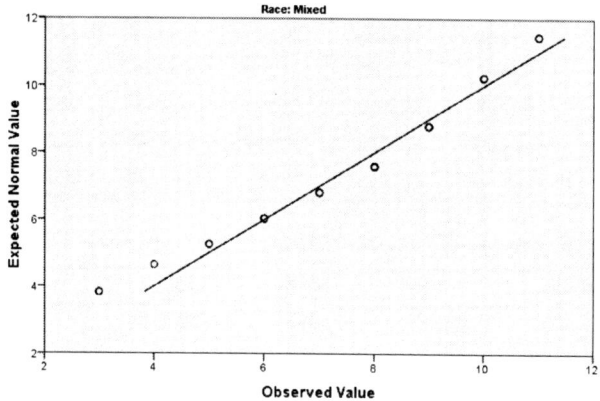

Figure 5.30 Correct attitude/perception of HIV and AIDS (Mixed) – normal Q-Q plot

Table 5.15 Descriptive Statistics of Ethnic Groups' Attitudes/Perceptions

	African	Indian	Chinese	Amer-indian	Portuguese	Mixed
Valid	154.000	146.000	6.000	15.000	10.000	48.000
Missing	.000	.000	.000	.000	.000	.000
Mean	8.156	7.575	5.000	8.067	6.600	7.646
Std. Error of Mean	.143	.180	1.238	.396	.686	.301
Median	8.000	8.000	5.000	8.000	7.000	8.000
Mode	8.000	8.000	3.000[a]	8.000	7.000	9.000
Std. Deviation	1.775	2.175	3.033	1.534	2.171	2.088
Variance	3.152	4.729	9.200	2.352	4.711	4.361
Skewness	−.551	−.236	−.194	.558	−1.147	−.602
Std. Error of Skewness	.195	.201	.845	.580	.687	.343
Kurtosis	.182	−.228	−2.396	−.639	1.206	−.204
Std. Error of Kurtosis	.389	.399	1.741	1.121	1.334	.674

Table 5.15 Descriptive Statistics of Ethnic Groups' Attitudes/Perceptions (continued)

	African	Indian	Chinese	Amer-indian	Portuguese	Mixed
Range	9.000	11.000	7.000	5.000	7.000	8.000
Minimum	2.000	1.000	1.000	6.000	2.000	3.000
Maximum	11.000	12.000	8.000	11.000	9.000	11.000
Sum	1256.000	1106.000	30.000	121.000	66.000	367.000

Table 5.16 Levene F Test on Attitudes/Perceptions – Ethnic Groups

Levene Statistic	df1	df2	Sig.
2.694	5	373	.021

ANOVA

Positive Attitudes/ Perceptions	Sum of Squares	df	Mean Square	F	Sig.
Between Groups	90.242	5	18.048	4.505	.001
Within Groups	1494.243	373	4.006		
Total	1584.485	378			

Table 5.17 Kruskal-Wallis Test Statistics[a,b] (Overall) on Ethnic Groups' Attitudes/Perceptions

	Positive Attitudes/Perceptions
Chi-Square	14.775
df	5
Asymp. Sig.	.011

a. Kruskal-Wallis Test

b. Grouping Variable: Ethnic Group

Table 5.18 Kruskal-Wallis Test Statistics[a,b] (Per Item) on Ethnic Groups' Attitudes/Perceptions

	Death	Punishment	Crime	Happens to Others	Horror	Jokes	Gossip
Chi-square	12.844	3.347	10.970	3.641	4.378	4.460	2.908
Df	5	5	5	5	5	5	5
Asymp. Sig.	.025	.647	.052	.602	.496	.485	.714

	Not Work	Not Sell Food	Not Comfortable	Not Sharing Work Tools	Not Sharing Toilet	Sitting Next to Person
Chi-square	2.045	3.243	8.854	17.095	17.573	7.001
Df	5	5	5	5	5	5
Asymp. Sig.	.843	.663	.115	.004	.004	.221

a. Kruskal-Wallis Test

b. Grouping Variable: Ethnic Group

Table 5.19 High School Students Paired by Ethnicity

Stigma-related Attitude/Perception Items	High School Students Paired by Ethnicity
1. HIV and AIDS is death.	African and Mixed
2. I would not be comfortable sharing work tools with an HIV- or AIDS-infected person.	African and Chinese; Indian and Chinese
3. I would not be comfortable sharing the toilet with an HIV- or AIDS-infected person.	African and Chinese; Amerindian and Chinese

Chapter 6

Predictors of Knowledge and Stigma-related Attitudes/ Perceptions

HIV and AIDS Knowledge

The bivariate analyses show that age, religion and ethnicity have a statistically significant relationship with the desired score for knowledge of HIV and AIDS, and that gender has no statistical significance with knowledge of HIV and AIDS. For this reason, gender was dropped from the multivariate analyses. Here, it is important to identify potential confounding variables (age, religion and ethnicity) and their relationship with knowledge of HIV and AIDS. In essence, variables that are predictors of correct knowledge of HIV and AIDS will be determined and discussed.

Since knowledge as the outcome of interest is dichotomous, the statistical procedure applied to identify multiple confounding variables, and thereby determine predictors of HIV and AIDS knowledge, is the multiple logistic regression model. This procedure can identify confounding variables because it examines all the explanatory variables simultaneously. The multiple logistic regression model was used to predict the probability of students having correct knowledge of HIV and AIDS over the probability of students not having correct knowledge of HIV and AIDS. Predictions are made with respect to the odds of students having low scores for knowledge of HIV and AIDS (0) compared to the likelihood of them having high scores for knowledge of HIV and AIDS (1). The logistic regression results for the full model on HIV and AIDS knowledge are in appendix 6. In the data given below, the author used odds ratio (OR) and confidence interval

(CI). OR indicates that students from particular religious and ethnic origins are less likely to have incorrect HIV and AIDS knowledge than those students coming from other religious and ethnic origins. CI is an interval calculated from sample data, and indicates the probability (90%, 95% and 99%) that the odds ratio is within the interval.

Age, religion and ethnicity are variables included in the full logistic regression model to determine whether they are predictors of correct knowledge of HIV and AIDS. The p-value of deviance of goodness of the fit chi-square test is 0.9618, which is greater than $\alpha = 0.05$. Therefore, it can be concluded that this model sufficiently fits the data. This means that the full logistic model can determine the number of students who scored correctly on the HIV and AIDS knowledge items and the number of students who scored incorrectly. This model also shows the coefficients, the Z estimates, p-values, odds ratios and confidence intervals for every predictor variable. These indicators suggest that all the religious groups (Christians, Hindus, Muslims and Others) and one ethnic group (Mixed) are statistically significant predictors of overall correct response for knowledge of HIV and AIDS and that there are also differences among them in their average scores. Nevertheless, these coefficients are negative, indicating that the religious groups and the Mixed ethnic group are associated with a less favourable overall score for knowledge of HIV and AIDS. Religious Group 2 (Hindus) has the strongest negative relationship with overall score ($b3 = -0.756398$) for knowledge of HIV and AIDS, and Religious Group 1 (Christians) has the weakest negative relationship with overall score ($b2 = -0.338755$) for knowledge of HIV and AIDS. For this reason, when compared to the other religious groups, Religious Group 1 obtained the most favourable overall score for knowledge of HIV and AIDS.

Overall, in the full model, controlling for other variables, the odds of students having incorrect knowledge of HIV/AIDS

- decrease by a factor of 0.712 if the student is from Religious Group 1 Christian (OR = 0.712657, CI 0.561711 to 0.904167);
- decrease by a factor of 0.469 if the student is from Religious Group 2 Hindu (OR = 0.469354, CI 0.328604 to 0.670391);
- decrease by a factor of 0.643 if the student is from Religious Group 3 Muslim (OR = 0.643741, CI 0.42886 to 0.966289);
- decrease by a factor of 0.686 if the student is from Religious Group 4 Other (OR = 0.686496, CI 0.493402 to 0.955157);
- decrease by a factor of 0.632 if the student is from Ethnic Group 6 Mixed (OR = 0.632431, CI 0.397142 to 1.007119).

This full model shows the following:

- that more Christian students than students from other religious groups have correct knowledge of HIV and AIDS; and
- that more ethnically mixed students than students from other ethnic groups have correct knowledge of HIV and AIDS.

All the predictor variables in the model (age, religion and ethnicity) are statistically significant except age; however, all the categories of each predictor variable are not statistically significant. For instance, being an African, Indian, Amerindian, Chinese or Portuguese student does not significantly impact the odds of such a student having low scores for the knowledge items on HIV and AIDS.

The Ten HIV and AIDS Knowledge Items

The same statistical procedure was used to examine each of the ten knowledge items (on the HIV and AIDS Knowledge Questionnaire) and their relationship with demographics (age, religion and ethnicity) as the predictor variables. The relevant data are in appendix 7.

The deviance of goodness of the fit chi-square value is 2.086713, and since the p-value of 0.9999 is greater than $\alpha = 0.05$, it can be concluded that the model fits the data correctly. This means, that in relation to Item 1 (the negative impact of HIV and AIDS on the immune system), this model can determine which students have correct knowledge, and which do not. Religious Groups 1, 2, 3 and 4 (Christians, Hindus, Muslims and Others) and Ethnic Group 1 (Africans) are statistically significant predictors of correct knowledge of the negative impact of HIV and AIDS on the immune system, but there are differences in their average scores.

Controlling for other variables, the odds of students having incorrect knowledge of item 1

- decrease by a factor of 0.717 if the student is from Religious Group 1 Christian (OR = .717, CI 0.590407 to 0.872836);
- decrease by a factor of 0.708 if the student is from Religious Group 2 Hindu (OR = .708, CI 0.545682 to 0.918652);
- decrease by a factor of 0.700 if the student is from Religious Group 3 Muslim (OR = .700, CI 0.501677 to 0.978914;
- decrease by a factor of 0.732 if the student is from Religious Group 4 Other (OR = 0.732926, CI 0.555391 to 0.967212); and
- decrease by a factor of 0.742 if the student is from Ethnic Group 1 African (OR = 0.74263, CI 0.571664 to 0.964727).

These results show the following:

- that the higher the number of students in religious groups, the higher the chances of correct knowledge of the negative impact of HIV and AIDS on the immune system; and
- that more African students than students from other ethnic groups have correct knowledge of the negative impact of HIV and AIDS on the immune system.

With regard to item 2 (symptoms of HIV and AIDS), the deviance of goodness of the fit is not statistically significant (chi square = 3.603058; p-value > 0.9999, which is greater than α = 0.05). The model, therefore, fits the data correctly. Religious Groups 1, 3 and 4 (Christians, Muslims and Others) and Ethnic Group 2 (Indians) are statistically significant predictors of correct knowledge of the symptoms of HIV and AIDS.

Furthermore, controlling for other variables, the odds of students having incorrect knowledge of item 2

- decrease by a factor of 0.623 if the student is from Religious Group 1 Christian (OR = 0.623373, CI 0.511811 to 0.759253);
- decrease by a factor of 0.696 if the student is from Religious Group 3 Muslim (OR = 0.696332, CI 0.499377 to 0.970968);
- decrease by a factor of 0.694 if the student is from Religious Group 4 Other (OR = 0.694568, CI 0.526353 to 0.916541); and
- decrease by a factor of 0.761 if the student is from Ethnic Group 2 Indian (OR = 0.761433, CI 0.578914 to 1.001496).

These results suggest the following:

- that more Muslim and Other (non-Christian and non-Hindu) students than students from other religious groups have correct knowledge of the symptoms of HIV and AIDS; and
- that more Indian students than students from other ethnic groups have correct knowledge of the symptoms of HIV and AIDS.

Pertaining to item 3 (HIV transmission vis-à-vis casual contact), the deviance of goodness of the fit is not statistically significant (chi square = 25.839242; p-value = 0.4162, which is greater than α = 0.05). The model, therefore, fits the data accurately. However, none of the predictor variables is statistically significant to predict correct knowledge of HIV and AIDS transmission vis-à-vis casual contact.

Concerning item 4 (HIV transmission through the normative methods), the deviance of goodness of the fit is not statistically significant (chi square = 3.428073; p-value > 0.9999, which is greater than $\alpha = 0.05$). The model, therefore, fits the data correctly. Religious Groups 1, 3 and 4 (Christians, Muslims and Others) and Ethnic Groups 1 and 2 (Africans and Indians) are statistically significant predictors of correct knowledge of HIV transmission through the normative methods.

Additionally, controlling for other variables, the odds of students having incorrect knowledge of item 4

- decrease by a factor of 0.653 if the student is from Religious Group 1 Christian (OR = 0.653616, CI 0.538317 to 0.793609);
- decrease by a factor of 0.696 if the student is from Religious Group 3 Muslim (OR = 0.696942, CI 0.501838 to 0.9679);
- decrease by a factor of 0.665 if the student is from Religious Group 4 Other (OR = 0.665494, CI 0.503994 to 0.87874);
- decrease by a factor of 0.759 if the student is from Ethnic Group 1 African (OR = 0.759427, CI 0.584623 to 0.986497); and
- decrease by a factor of 0.754 if the student is from Ethnic Group 2 Indian (OR = 0.754817, CI 0.577325 to 0.986876).

These results suggest the following:

- that more Muslim students than students from other religious groups have correct knowledge of HIV transmission through the normative methods; and
- that more African and Indian students than students from other ethnic groups have correct knowledge of HIV transmission through the normative methods.

As it relates to item 5 (the non-transmission of HIV vis-à-vis coughing, sneezing, etc.), the deviance of goodness of the fit is not statistically significant (chi square = 9.242283; p-value = 0.9982, which is greater than $\alpha = 0.05$). Therefore, the model fits the data well. Religious Groups 1, 3 and 4 (Christians, Muslims and Others) and Ethnic Groups 1 and 2 (Africans and Indians) are statistically significant predictors of correct knowledge of the non-transmission of HIV vis-à-vis coughing, sneezing, etc.

Moreover, controlling for other variables, the odds of students having incorrect knowledge of item 5

- decrease by a factor of 0.662 if the student is from Religious Group 1 Christian (OR = 0.662421, CI 0.537158 to 0.816897);
- decrease by a factor of 0.663 if the student is from Religious Group 3 Muslim (OR = 0.663151, CI0.46269 to 0.950462);

- decrease by a factor of 0.631 if the student is from Religious Group 4 Other (OR = 0.631956, CI 0.466176 to 0.85669);
- decrease by a factor of 0.688 if the student is from Ethnic Group 1 African (OR = 0.688886, CI 0.523068 to 0.90727); and
- decrease by a factor of 0.664 if the student is from Ethnic Group 2 Indian (OR = 0.664578, CI 0.499857 to 0.883581).

These results suggest the following:

- that more Muslim, Christian and Other students than Hindu students have correct knowledge of the non-transmission of HIV vis-à-vis coughing, sneezing, etc.; and
- that more African and Indian students than students of other ethnic groups have correct knowledge of the non-transmission of HIV vis-à-vis coughing, sneezing, etc.

Regarding item 6 (the asymptomatic nature of HIV and AIDS), the deviance of goodness of the fit is not statistically significant (chi square=5.13065; p-value >0.9999, which is greater than $\alpha = 0.05$). Therefore, the model fits the data accurately. Only the religious groups are statistically significant predictors of correct knowledge of the asymptomatic nature of HIV and AIDS.

Furthermore, controlling for other variables, the odds of students having incorrect knowledge of item 6

- decrease by a factor of 0.679 if the student is from Religious Group 1 Christian (OR = 0.67965, CI 0.552831 to 0.835561);
- decrease by a factor of 0.706 if the student is from Religious Group 2 Hindu (OR = 0.706122, CI 0.536513 to 0.929349);
- decrease by a factor of 0.659 if the student is from Religious Group 3 Muslim (OR = 0.659634, CI 0.462244 to 0.941316); and
- decrease by a factor of 0.731 if the student is from Religious Group 4 Other (OR = 0.731803, CI 0.5486 to 0.976187).

These results indicate the following:

- that all the religious groups have correct knowledge of the asymptomatic nature of HIV and AIDS; and
- that all the ethnic groups as predictor variables in the model are not statistically significant. For instance, being an African, Indian, Amerindian, Chinese or Portuguese student does not impact significantly the odds of such a student having incorrect knowledge of the asymptomatic nature of HIV and AIDS.

With respect to item 7 (the non-transmission of HIV through blood donation), the deviance of goodness of the fit is not statistically significant (chi square = 23.570029; p-value = 0.5443, which is greater than α = 0.05). Therefore, the model fits the data quite well. Only Religious Groups 1, 2 and 3 (Christians, Hindus and Muslims) are statistically significant predictors of correct knowledge of the non-transmission of HIV through blood donation.

Furthermore, controlling for other variables, the odds of students having incorrect knowledge of item 7

- decrease by a factor of 0.688 if the student is from Religious Group 1 Christian (OR = 0.688553, CI 0.523491 to 0.90566);
- decrease by a factor of 0.467 if the student is from Religious Group 2 Hindu (OR = 0.467806, CI 0.316682 to 0.691048); and
- decrease by a factor of 0.465 if the student is from Religious Group 3 Muslim (OR = 0.465625, CI 0.276314 to 0.78464).

These results indicate the following:

- that Christian students more than students from other religious groups have correct knowledge of the non-transmission of HIV through blood donation; and
- that all the ethnic groups as predictor variables in the model are not statistically significant. For instance, being an African, Indian, Amerindian, Chinese or Portuguese student does not impact significantly the odds of such a student having incorrect knowledge of the non-transmission of HIV through blood donation.

With regard to item 8 (the non-transmission of HIV vis-à-vis mosquitoes and domesticated animals), the deviance of goodness of the fit is not statistically significant (chi square = 28.425225; p-value = 0.2887, which is greater than α = 0.05). Therefore, the model fits the data accurately. With the exception of age, none of the predictor variables is statistically significant to predict correct knowledge of the non- transmission of HIV vis-à-vis mosquitoes and domesticated animals.

Furthermore, controlling for other variables, the likelihood of students not having correct knowledge of item 8

- decreases by a factor of 0.571 if the student is from the higher age group (OR = 0.571672, CI 0.343298 to 0.951969).

This result shows that all the religious and ethnic groups as predictor variables in the model are not statistically significant. For instance, being a

Christian, Hindu, Muslim or Other; and being an African, Indian, Amerindian, Chinese or Portuguese student does not impact significantly the odds of such a student having incorrect knowledge of the non-transmission of HIV vis-à-vis mosquitoes and domesticated animals.

Concerning item 9 (the improbability of contracting HIV by being around an HIV-infected person), the deviance of goodness of the fit is not statistically significant (chi square = 24.928145; p-value = 0.4097, which is greater than α = 0.05). Therefore, the model fits the data correctly. None of the predictor variables is statistically significant to predict correct knowledge of the improbability of contracting HIV by being around an HIV-infected person. This result indicates that the students from the various religious groups, ethnic groups and age groups show no differences in their response to item 9.

Finally, with reference to item 10 (the need to institute preventive measures against contracting HIV), the deviance of goodness of the fit is not statistically significant (chi square = 6.134932; p-value = 0.9999, which is greater than α = 0.05). Therefore, the model fits the data quite well. Religious Groups 1, 2, 3 and 4 (Christians, Hindus, Muslims and Others) and Ethnic Groups 2 and 6 (Indians and Mixed) are statistically significant predictors of correct knowledge of the need to institute preventive measures against contracting HIV.

Furthermore, controlling for other variables, the odds of students having incorrect knowledge of item 10

- decrease by a factor of 0.753 if the student is from Religious Group 1 Christian (OR = 0.753249, CI 0.602235 to 0.942132);
- decrease by a factor of 0.661 if the student is from Religious Group 2 Hindu (OR = 0.661074, CI 0.482463 to 0.90581);
- decrease by a factor of 0.683 if the student is from Religious Group 3 Muslim (OR = 0.683901, CI 0.462189 to 1.011967);
- decrease by a factor of 0.683 if the student is from Religious Group 4 Other (OR = 0.683178, CI 0.496019 to 0.940955);
- decrease by a factor of 0.712 if the student is from Ethnic Group 2 Indian (OR = 0.712609, CI 0.523927 to 0.96924); and
- decrease by a factor of 0.559 if the student is from Ethnic Group 6 Mixed (OR = 0.559613, CI 0.365497 to 0.856824).

The results show that Christian and Indian students more than other students have correct knowledge as it relates to the need to institute preventive measures against contracting HIV.

In the full model of the logistic regression analysis, religion and ethnicity as variables are statistically significant (p < 0.05), and they are predictors of HIV and AIDS knowledge. Age as a variable is not statistically significant, and, therefore, is not a predictor of knowledge. Identifying the predictors of HIV and AIDS stigma-related attitudes/perceptions is the next step, prior to determining the relationship between HIV and AIDS knowledge and stigma-related attitudes/perceptions.

HIV and AIDS Stigma-related Attitudes and Perceptions

The bivariate analyses show that gender and age have no association with appropriate attitudes/perceptions of HIV and AIDS, and, therefore, were dropped from the multivariate analysis. However, religion and ethnicity have a statistically significant relationship with appropriate attitudes/ perceptions of HIV and AIDS.

It is important to identify potential confounding variables (religion and ethnicity) in their relationship with HIV and AIDS stigma-related attitudes/perceptions, that is, it is essential to determine which variables influence the development of appropriate perceptions/attitudes toward PLHIV and which do not. Since appropriate attitudes/perceptions as the outcome of interest are dichotomous, the statistical procedure to establish this identification is the multiple logistic regression model. This procedure can identify the confounding variables because it examines all the explanatory variables simultaneously.

It is predicted that the likelihood of high school students having appropriate perceptions/attitudes toward PLHIV is related to the students' religion and/or ethnicity. Predictions are also made with respect to the odds of students having low scores for the HIV and AIDS attitude/perception items (0) compared to the likelihood of them having high scores for the HIV and AIDS attitude/perception items (1). The logistic regression results for the full model are in appendix 8.

Another main interest in this study is to determine whether religion and ethnicity are predictors of positive HIV and AIDS attitudes/perceptions. The p-value of deviance of goodness of the fit chi-square test is 0.9542, which is greater than $\alpha = 0.05$. It can, therefore, be concluded that the model fits the data correctly. This means that this full model can determine the number of students who scored correctly on the HIV and AIDS attitude/perception items and the number of students who scored incorrectly. This model also shows the coefficients, the Z estimates, p-values, odds ratios and confidence intervals for both predictor variables – Religious Groups and Ethnic Groups. These indicators suggest that all the Religious Groups are statistically significant predictors of overall high score for correct response to the HIV and AIDS attitude/perception items, but there are also differences in the groups' mean scores.

Controlling for other variables, the odds of students having inappropriate attitudes/perceptions of HIV and AIDS

- decrease by a factor of 0.644 if the student is from Religious Group 1 Christian (OR = 0.644868, CI 0.509388 to 0.816381);
- decrease by a factor of 0.514 if the student is from Religious Group 2 Hindu (OR = 0.514666, CI 0.371931 to 0.712178);
- decrease by a factor of 0.695 if the student is from Religious Group 3 Muslim (OR = 0.695241, CI 0.484705 to 0.997226); and
- decrease by a factor of 0.676 if the student is from Religious Group 4 Other (OR = 0.676232, CI 0.490564 to 0.932171).

These results suggest that in the full model

- the Muslim and Other students more than the Hindu and Christian students have appropriate attitudes/perceptions of HIV and AIDS; and
- the ethnic groups as predictor variables are not statistically significant. For instance, being an African, Indian, Amerindian, Chinese or Portuguese student does not impact significantly the odds of such a student having inappropriate attitudes/perceptions of HIV and AIDS.

The Thirteen HIV and AIDS Stigma-related Attitude/Perception Items

The same statistical procedure was used to examine each of the thirteen stigma-related attitude/perception items (on the HIV and AIDS Stigma-related Attitudes/Perceptions Questionnaire) and their relationships with the demographic variables (religion and ethnicity) as predictors. The relevant data are in appendix 9.

The deviance of goodness of the fit chi-square value is 9.391207, and since the p-value of 0.6692 is greater than $\alpha = 0.05$, it can be concluded that the model fits the data correctly. This means that in relation to item 1 (HIV and AIDS is death), this model can determine the number of students who scored correctly on this item and the number of students who scored incorrectly. Religious Groups 1, 3 and 4 (Christians, Muslims and Others) and Ethnic Group 1 (Africans) are statistically significant predictors of appropriate attitude/perception of HIV and AIDS in relation to the idea expressed in item 1. It is important to note, however, that differences exist in the groups' average scores.

Controlling for other variables, the odds of students having an inappropriate attitude/perception in relation to the idea expressed in item 1

- decrease by a factor of 0.590 if the student is from Religious Group 1 Christian (OR = 0.590231, CI 0.466678 to 0.746493);
- decrease by a factor of 0.550 if the student is from Religious Group 3 Muslim (OR = 0.550749, CI 0.378027 to 0.802387);
- decrease by a factor of 0.736 if the student is from Religious Group 4 Other (OR = 0.736983, CI 0.538234 to 1.009121); and
- decrease by a factor of 0.574 if the student is from Ethnic Group 1 African (OR = 0.57484, CI 0.41224 to 0.801575).

These results show the following:

- that students from Other religious groups more than those from the Christian, Hindu and Muslim groups have the appropriate attitude/perception of HIV and AIDS with respect to item 1; and
- that there are no differences in the appropriate attitude/perception of HIV and AIDS among African, Indian, Mixed, Chinese, Portuguese and Amerindian students, as Ethnic Groups as predictor variables are not significant.

With regard to item 2 (HIV and AIDS is punishment), the deviance of goodness of the fit is not statistically significant (chi square = 6.284508; p-value > 0.9011, which is greater than $\alpha = 0.05$). The model, therefore, is exact. Religious Groups 1, 3 and 4 (Christians, Muslims and Others) and Ethnic Groups 1, 2 and 6 (Africans, Indians and Mixed) are statistically significant predictors of appropriate attitude/perception of HIV and AIDS in relation to the opinion expressed in item 2.

Furthermore, controlling for other variables, the odds of students having an inappropriate attitude/perception in relation to the idea expressed in item 2

- decrease by a factor of 0.546 if the student is from Religious Group 1 Christian (OR = 0.546006, CI 0.421059 to 0.708031);
- decrease by a factor of 0.582 if the student is from Religious Group 3 Muslim (OR = 0.582205, CI 0.3884 to 0.872715);
- decrease by a factor of 0.680 if the student is from Religious Group 4 Other (OR = 0.680933, CI 0.482129 to 0.961713);
- decrease by a factor of 0.585 if the student is from Ethnic Group 1 African (OR = 0.585526, CI 0.417294 to 0.821581);

- decrease by a factor of 0.622 if the student is from Ethnic Group 2 Indian (OR = 0.622945, CI 0.440893 to 0.88017);
- decrease by a factor of 0.569 if the student is from Ethnic Group 6 Mixed (OR = 0.569017, CI 0.365133 to 0.886745).

These results show the following:

- that students from Other religious groups more than students from the remaining religious groups have an appropriate attitude/perception of HIV and AIDS with respect to item 2; and
- that Indian students more than students from other ethnic groups have an appropriate attitude/perception of HIV and AIDS with respect to item 2.

Pertaining to item 3 (HIV and AIDS is a crime), the deviance of goodness of the fit is statistically significant (chi square = 23.435438; p-value = 0.0242, which is less than $\alpha = 0.05$). The model, therefore, is not a good fit of the data. In addition, none of the predictor variables is statistically significant to predict appropriate attitude/perception of HIV and AIDS as it relates to item 3. At any rate, the predictor coefficients not being statistically significant indicate that there are no differences in the religious and ethnic groups' view of the idea expressed in item 3.

Concerning item 4 (HIV and AIDS only happen to others), the deviance of goodness of the fit is not statistically significant (chi square = 10.723329; p-value = 0.5528, which is greater than $\alpha = 0.05$). The model, therefore, fits the data correctly. Nevertheless, none of the predictor variables is statistically significant to predict appropriate attitude/perception of HIV and AIDS as it relates to item 4. In effect, religion and ethnicity are not good predictors of the perception that HIV and AIDS only happen to others.

Regarding item 5 (HIV and AIDS is horror), the deviance of goodness of the fit is not statistically significant (chi square =8.889519; p-value= 0.7123, which is greater than $\alpha = 0.05$). Therefore, the model fits the data quite well. Religious Groups 1, 3 and 4 (Christians, Muslims and Others) and Ethnic Groups 1, 2 and 6 (Africans, Indians and Mixed) are statistically significant predictors of appropriate attitude/perception of HIV and AIDS in relation to the idea expressed in item 5.

Moreover, controlling for other variables, the odds of students having an inappropriate attitude/perception in relation to the idea expressed in item 5

- decrease by a factor of 0.631 if the student is from Religious Group 1 Christian (OR=0.63115, CI 0.502047 to 0.793453);

- decrease by a factor of 0.609 if the student is from Religious Group 3 Muslim (OR=0.609102, CI 0.421474 to 0.880258);
- decrease by a factor of 0.668 if the student is from Religious Group 4 Other (OR=0.668962, CI 0.486648 to 0.919576);
- decrease by a factor of 0.614 if the student is from Ethnic Group 1 African (OR=0.614242, CI 0.457193 to 0.82524);
- decrease by a factor of 0.574 if the student is from Ethnic Group 2 Indian (OR=0.574792, CI 0.421076 to 0.784622); and
- decrease by a factor of 0.623 if the student is from Ethnic Group 6 Mixed (OR=0.623533, CI 0.425254 to 0.914263).

These results indicate the following:

- that students from the Other religious groups more than students from the remaining religious groups have an appropriate attitude/perception of HIV and AIDS with respect to item 5; and
- that African and mixed-race students more than Indian students have an appropriate attitude/perception of HIV and AIDS with respect to item 5.

With regard to item 6 (People make jokes about PLHIV), the deviance of goodness of the fit is not statistically significant (chi square = 5.485809; p-value = 0.9398, which is greater than $\alpha = 0.05$). Therefore, the model fits the data quite well. All the Religious Groups (Christians, Muslims, Hindus and Others) and Ethnic Groups 1 and 2 (Africans and Indians) are statistically significant predictors of appropriate attitude/perception of PLHIV in relation to the idea expressed in item 6.

Moreover, controlling for other variables, the odds of students having an inappropriate attitude/perception in relation to the idea expressed in item 6

- decrease by a factor of 0.703 if the student is from Religious Group 1 Christian (OR = 0.70383, CI 0.580281 to 0.853684);
- decrease by a factor of 0.740 if the student is from Religious Group 2 Hindu (OR = 0.740872, CI 0.578371 to 0.94903);
- decrease by a factor of 0.680 if the student is from Religious Group 3 Muslim (OR = 0.680392, CI 0.501799 to 0.922547);
- decrease by a factor of 0.749 if the student is from Religious Group 4 Other (OR = 0.749493, CI 0.574368 to 0.978013);
- decrease by a factor of 0.633 if the student is from Ethnic Group 1 African (OR = 0.633, CI 0.487518 to 0.821897); and
- decrease by a factor of 0.700 if the student is from Ethnic Group 2 Indian (OR = 0.700268, CI 0.534452 to 0.917529).

These results show the following:

- that among the religious groups, the Hindu, Other and Christian students have the most appropriate attitude/perception of PLHIV with respect to item 6; and
- that Indian more than African students have an appropriate attitude/perception of PLHIV with respect to item 6.

With reference to item 7 (People gossip about PLHIV), the deviance of goodness of the fit is not statistically significant (chi square = 2.053689; p-value = 0.9993, which is greater than α = 0.05). The model, therefore, fits the data accurately. Religious Groups 1, 3 and 4 (Christians, Muslims and Others) and Ethnic Groups 1, 2 and 6 (Africans, Indians and Mixed) are statistically significant predictors of appropriate attitude/perception of PLHIV in relation to the view expressed in item 7.

Furthermore, controlling for other variables, the odds of students having an inappropriate attitude/perception in relation to the idea expressed in item 7

- decrease by a factor of 0.676 if the student is from Religious Group 1 Christian (OR = 0.676421, CI 0.55872 to 0.818917);
- decrease by a factor of 0.686 if the student is from Religious Group 3 Muslim (OR = 0.686183, CI 0.508073 to 0.926732);
- decrease by a factor of 0.736 if the student is from Religious Group 4 Other (OR = 0.736709, CI 0.567037 to 0.957151);
- decrease by a factor of 0.706 if the student is from Ethnic Group 1 African (OR = 0.70693, CI 0.546241 to 0.91489);
- decrease by a factor of 0.692 if the student is from Ethnic Group 2 Indian (OR = 0.692429 CI 0.528836 to 0.906628); and
- decrease by a factor of 0.692 if the student is from Ethnic Group 6 Mixed (OR = 0.692303, CI 0.496019 to 0.966261).

These results indicate the following:

- that students from the Other religious groups more than those from the remaining religious groups have the most appropriate attitude/perception of PLHIV with respect to item 7; and
- that Africans, Indians and mixed-race students have the most appropriate attitude/perception of PLHIV with respect to item 7.

Pertaining to Item 8 (PLHIV should not gain employment), the deviance of goodness of the fit is not statistically significant (chi square = 9.054456; p-value = 0.6983, which is greater than α = 0.05). The model, therefore, is a good fit for the data. Nevertheless, none of the predictor variables is statistically significant to predict appropriate attitude/perception of PLHIV in relation to the belief expressed in item 8. No statistical significance indicates that there are any differences in the attitude/perception of the religious and ethnic groups as it relates to employment for PLHIV.

With regard to item 9 (PLHIV should not sell food), the deviance of goodness of fit is not statistically significant (chi square = 7.348326; p-value = 0.8338, which is greater than α = 0.05). The model, therefore, fits the data accurately. Religious Groups 1 and 3 (Christians and Muslims) and Ethnic Groups 1, 2 and 6 (Africans, Indians and Mixed) are significant predictors of appropriate attitude/perception of HIV and AIDS in relation to the view expressed in item 9.

Furthermore, controlling for other variables, the odds of students having an inappropriate attitude/perception in relation to the idea expressed in item 9

- decrease by a factor of 0.574 if the student is from Religious Group 1 Christian (OR = 0.574877, CI 0.422252 to 0.782669);
- decrease by a factor of 0.394 if the student is from Religious Group 3 Muslim (OR = 0.394663, CI 0.227307 to 0.685236);
- decrease by a factor of 0.498 if the student is from Ethnic Group 1 African (OR = 0.498148, CI 0.33804 to 0.734087);
- decrease by a factor of 0.567 if the student is from Ethnic Group 2 Indian (OR = 0.567868, CI 0.381809 to 0.844595); and
- decrease by a factor of 0.517 if the student is from Ethnic Group 6 Mixed (OR = 0.517387, CI 0.310652 to 0.861703).

These results suggest the following:

- that more Christian students than students from other religious groups have an appropriate attitude/perception of PLHIV with respect to item 9; and
- that more Indian students than students from other ethnic groups have an appropriate attitude/perception of PLHIV with respect to item 9.

With reference to item 10 (Uncomfortable shaking hands with PLHIV), the deviance of goodness of the fit is not statistically significant (chi square = 13.749782; p-value = 0.317, which is greater than α = 0.05). The model, therefore, fits the data correctly. Religious Groups 1 and 4 (Christians and Others) and Ethnic Groups 1, 2 and 6 (Africans, Indians and

Mixed) are significant predictors of appropriate attitude/perception of PLHIV in relation to the view expressed in item 10.

Furthermore, controlling for other variables, the odds of students having an inappropriate attitude/perception in relation to the idea expressed in item 10

- decrease by a factor of 0.423 if the student is from Religious Group 1 Christian (OR = 0.423934, CI 0.287195 to 0.625777);
- decrease by a factor of 0.578 if the student is from Religious Group 4 Other (OR = 0.578396, CI 0.346834 to 0.96456);
- decrease by a factor of 0.480 if the student is from Ethnic Group 1 African (OR = 0.480507, CI0.298001 to 0.774788);
- decrease by a factor of 0.642 if the student is from Ethnic Group 2 Indian (OR = 0.642975, CI 0.393663 to 1.050182; and
- decrease by a factor of 0.486 if the student is from Ethnic Group 6 Mixed (OR = 0.486883, CI 0.260227 to 0.910956).

These results suggest the following:

- that more students from Other religious groups than students from the remaining religious groups have an appropriate attitude/perception of PLHIV with respect to item 10; and
- that more Indian students than students from other ethnic groups have an appropriate attitude/perception of PLHIV with respect to item 10.

Pertaining to item 11 (Uncomfortable sharing work tools with PLHIV), the deviance of goodness of the fit is not statistically significant (chi square=17.57212; p-value= 0.1293, which is greater than α = 0.05). The model, therefore, is a good fit for the data. Nevertheless, none of the predictor variables is statistically significant to predict appropriate attitude/perception of PLHIV in relation to the belief expressed in item 11. At any rate, no statistical significance indicates that there are any differences in the attitude/perception of the religious and ethnic groups as it relates to sharing work tools with PLHIV.

With regard to item 12 (Uncomfortable sharing toilet facilities with PLHIV), the deviance of goodness of the fit is not statistically significant (chi square = 8.75289; p-value = 0.7239, which is greater than α = 0.05). The model, therefore, fits the data correctly. Religious Groups 1, 3 and 4 (Christians, Muslims and Others) and Ethnic Groups 1, 2, 3, 4 and 6 (Africans, Indians, Chinese, Amerindians and Mixed) are significant predictors of appropriate attitude/perception of PLHIV in relation to sharing toilet facilities with PLHIV.

Furthermore, controlling for other variables, the odds of students having an inappropriate attitude/perception in relation to the idea expressed in item 12

- decrease by a factor of 0.460 if the student is from Religious Group 1 Christian (OR = 0.460412, CI 0.328054 to 0.64617);
- decrease by a factor of 0.536 if the student is from Religious Group 3 Muslim (OR = 0.536796, CI 0.320804 to 0.898211);
- decrease by a factor of 0.497 if the student is from Religious Group 4 Other (OR = 0.497143, CI 0.307825 to 0.802893);
- decrease by a factor of 0.496 if the student is from Ethnic Group 1 African (OR = 0.496453, CI 0.319511 to 0.771383);
- decrease by a factor of 0.534 if the student is from Ethnic Group 2 Indian (OR = 0.534473, CI 0.345875 to 0.82591);
- decrease by a factor of 3.219 if the student is from Ethnic Group 3 Chinese (OR = 3.219935, CI 1.348878 to 7.686375);
- decrease by a factor of 0.264 if the student is from Ethnic Group 4 Amerindian (OR = 0.264936 CI 0.0777 to 0.903364); and
- decrease by a factor of 0.472 if the student is from Ethnic Group 6 Mixed (OR = 0.472488, CI 0.270577 to 0.82507).

These results show the following:

- that more Muslim students than students from other religious groups have an appropriate attitude/perception of PLHIV with respect to item 12; and
- that more Chinese and Indian students than students from other ethnic groups have an appropriate attitude/perception of PLHIV with respect to item 12.

Finally, concerning item 13 (Perceived HIV or AIDS status by association), the deviance of goodness of the fit is not statistically significant (chi square = 13.105579; p-value = 0.3614, which is greater than α = 0.05). The model, therefore, fits the data correctly. Religious Groups 1, 3 and 4 (Christians, Muslims and Others) and Ethnic Groups 1, 2, 3 and 6 (Africans, Indians, Chinese and Mixed) are significant predictors of appropriate attitude/perception of PLHIV in relation to item 13.

Furthermore, controlling for other variables, the odds of students having an inappropriate attitude/perception in relation to the idea expressed in item 13

- decrease by a factor of 0.706 if the student is from Religious Group 1 Christian (OR = 0.706517, CI 0.539742 to 0.924824);
- decrease by a factor of 0.395 if the student is from Religious Group 3 Muslim (OR = 0.395491, CI 0.239681 to 0.652589);
- decrease by a factor of 0.679 if the student is from Religious Group 4 Other (OR = 0.67992, CI 0.46719 to 0.989514);
- decrease by a factor of 0.505 if the student is from Ethnic Group 1 African (OR = 0.505362, CI 0.361801 to 0.705888);
- decrease by a factor of 0.606 if the student is from Ethnic Group 2 Indian (OR = 0.606261, CI 0.428732 to 0.8573);
- decrease by a factor of 1.876 if the student is from Ethnic Group 3 Chinese (OR = 3.219935, CI 1.348878 to 7.686375;
- decrease by a factor of 0.504 if the student is from Ethnic Group 6 Mixed (OR = 0.50436CI 0.320593 to 0.793473).

These results indicate the following:

- that more Christian and Other students than Hindu and Muslim students have an appropriate attitude/perception of PLHIV with respect to item 13, that is, more Hindu and Muslim students perceive HIV or AIDS status by association than Christian and Other students;
- that more Chinese and Indian students than students from other ethnic groups have an appropriate attitude/perception of PLHIV with respect to item 13.

Relationship between HIV and AIDS Knowledge and Stigma-related Attitudes/ Perceptions

Appendix 10 provides the results on the analysis of the logistic regression for each HIV and AIDS knowledge (Predictor) question (1–10 together) and one item at a time on HIV and AIDS stigma-related attitudes (Response).

This table shows the odds ratios (OR) and 95% confidence intervals (CI) of HIV and AIDS knowledge variables as predictors associated with HIV and AIDS stigma-related attitudes (HIV and AIDS is death; HIV and AIDS is a crime; and uneasiness to share toilet facilities with PLHIV).

The belief that "HIV is not transmitted by sneezing, etc." (an indicator of HIV knowledge) is significantly associated with the view that "HIV and AIDS is death". High school students who know that a person cannot con-

Table 6.1 OR & 95% CI of Variables for HIV and AIDS Stigma-related Attitudes and Perceptions of PLHIV

Predictor HIV and AIDS Knowledge Variables	HIV and AIDS is Death	HIV and AIDS is a Crime	Uneasy to share toilet facilities with PLHIV
HIV is not transmitted by sneezing, etc.	0.441 (0.24–0.83) P = 0.01		
Testing HIV-positive does not signify the contraction of AIDS.		0.280 (0.09–0.85) P = 0.02	
Contracting HIV infection from insects and animals			2.67 (1.23–5.80) P = 0.01

tract HIV through sneezing, coughing, etc. (OR = 0.441221, 95% CI 0.24–0.83, p-value = 0.01) are less likely to view HIV and AIDS as death. When controlling for other variables, the odds of not having this relationship decrease by a factor of 0.441.

The idea that "Testing HIV-positive does not signify the contraction of AIDS" (an indicator of HIV and AIDS knowledge) is significantly associated with the belief that "HIV and AIDS is not a crime". High school students who know that a person who tested HIV-positive does not have AIDS (OR = 0.280172, 95% CI 0.09–0.85, p-value = 0.02) are less likely to view HIV and AIDS as a crime. When controlling for other variables, the odds of not having this relationship decrease by a factor of 0.280.

The view that "HIV infection can be contracted from insects and animals" (an indicator of HIV knowledge) is significantly associated with the "uneasiness to share toilet facilities with PLHIV". High school students who understand that a person cannot contract the HIV infection from insects and animals (OR = 2.67128, 95% CI 1.23–5.80, p-value = 0.01) are more likely to share toilet facilities with PLHIV. When controlling for other variables, the odds of not having this relationship decrease by a factor of 2.671.

Establishing students' knowledge of HIV and AIDS through "True/False" response on the following beliefs – "HIV is not transmitted by sneezing, etc"; "Testing HIV-positive does not signify the contraction of AIDS"; and "HIV infection can be contracted from insects and animals" – revealed students' misconceptions on transmission modes and HIV testing interpretations. These misconceptions and myths are some of the non-normative aspects. In this study, the results show that these three misconceptions are probable predictors of HIV and AIDS stigma-related attitudes/perceptions vis-à-vis their statistical significance. There were no associations between the other variables of HIV and AIDS knowledge and stigma-related attitudes/perceptions.

Chapter 7

Discussion and Implications

A study was conducted among high school students to compare differences in students' HIV and AIDS knowledge and stigma-related attitudes. A sample size of 379 students (39% aged 13–15 and 60% aged 16–18) participated in this research. The social composition of the sample comprised 42% males and 58% females. Of this group, 53% were Christians, 23% were Hindus and 10% were Muslims. Additionally, 40% of the sample population were Africans, 38% were Indians and 13% were mixed races.

The research questions in this study are as follows:

- What is the status of HIV and AIDS knowledge and stigma-related attitudes/perceptions among high school students?
- What are the differences in HIV and AIDS knowledge and stigma-related attitudes by gender, age, religious groups and ethnic groups?
- Is there an overall relationship between HIV and AIDS knowledge and stigma-related attitudes?
- Is there a relationship between the non-normative aspects of HIV and AIDS knowledge and stigma-related attitudes?

As the findings would indicate, this study has answered all the research questions. The findings are summarized as follows:

Univariate Findings
High School Students' Knowledge of HIV and AIDS

- On average, students showed moderate knowledge, scoring correctly on 7.47 items out of 10.

- 20% revealed misconceptions on HIV transmission, HIV testing interpretations and HIV prevention.
- 97.4% identified the modes of HIV transmission.
- 94.2% recognized the symptoms of HIV and AIDS.
- 55.9% indicated that a blood donor could contract HIV vis-à-vis blood
  donation.
- 30.1% indicated that there is need to institute preventive measures to
  protect oneself from the HIV infection.
- 60.1% of the female students and 56.5% of the male students revealed
  moderate knowledge of HIV and AIDS.
- 55.4% of the 13–15 age group and 68.6% of the 16–18 age group
  revealed moderate knowledge of HIV and AIDS.
- Christian (75.2%), Hindu (34%), Muslim (59.5%) and Other (71.2%)
  high school students exhibited moderate knowledge of HIV and AIDS.
- African (81.8%), Indian (52.7%), Chinese (50%), Amerindian
  (86.7%), Portuguese (40%) and Mixed (37.5%) high school students
  demonstrated moderate knowledge of HIV and AIDS.

High School Students' Attitudes/Perceptions of HIV and AIDS

- 60% indicated appropriate attitudes/perceptions of HIV, AIDS and
  PLHIV, and 40% indicated inappropriate attitudes/perceptions of
  HIV, AIDS and PLHIV.
- 94.2% indicated that if they had AIDS, people would call them names
  and gossip about them.
- 89.7% believed that people make jokes about people who are HIV-
  positive.
- 63.6% expressed the opinion that HIV and AIDS is horror.
- 59.4% conveyed the view that HIV and AIDS is death.
- 51.2% communicated the belief that HIV and AIDS is punishment.
- Students held these inappropriate attitudes/perceptions, notwithstanding their moderate knowledge of HIV and AIDS, suggesting that
  knowledge has minimum impact on attitudes/perceptions.
- 60.6% of the female students and 58.4% of the male students revealed
  appropriate attitudes/perceptions of HIV, AIDS and PLHIV.
- 59.5% of the 13–15 age group and 59.8% of the 16–18 age group
  revealed appropriate attitudes/perceptions of HIV, AIDS and PLHIV.
- Christian (61.9%), Hindu (54.5%), Muslim (62.2%) and Other
  (57.7%) students revealed appropriate attitudes/perceptions of HIV,
  AIDS and PLHIV.
- African (63%), Indian (58.3%), Chinese (38.3%), Amerindian (62%),
  Portuguese (51%) and Mixed (58.8%) students revealed appropriate
  attitudes/perceptions of HIV, AIDS and PLHIV.

Bivariate Findings
HIV and AIDS Knowledge

* There was no statistical significance in the mean score for HIV and AIDS knowledge of the male and female students.
* There was statistical significance in the mean score for HIV and AIDS knowledge of the 13–15 and 16–18 age groups.
* There was statistical significance in the median score for HIV and AIDS knowledge of the religious groups.
* There was statistical significance in the median score for HIV and AIDS knowledge of the ethnic groups.

HIV and AIDS Stigma-related Attitudes/Perceptions

* There was no statistical significance in the mean score for HIV and AIDS stigma-related attitudes/perceptions of male and female students.
* There was no statistical significance in the mean score for HIV and AIDS stigma-related attitudes/perceptions of the 13–15 and 16–18 age groups.
* There was statistical significance in the mean score for HIV and AIDS stigma-related attitudes of the religious groups.
* There was statistical significance in the median score for HIV and AIDS stigma-related attitudes of the ethnic groups.

Multiple Logistic Regression
HIV and AIDS Knowledge – The Full Model

* Religious groups and high scores for HIV and AIDS knowledge were statistically significant; religious groups were predictors of high scores for knowledge of HIV and AIDS.
* Ethnic groups and high scores for HIV and AIDS knowledge were not statistically significant.

All these predictor variables (religious groups) in the model were statistically significant. However, all the categories of each ethnic group (predictor) variable were not statistically significant. For instance, being an African, Indian, Amerindian, Chinese, Portuguese or mixed-race student did not impact significantly the odds of students having low scores for the knowledge items on HIV and AIDS. There was also no category of the predictor variables in the model that significantly increased the odds of students having low scores for the knowledge items on HIV and AIDS compared to their corresponding reference categories since there were no significant odds ratios greater than 1.

HIV and AIDS Stigma-related Attitudes/Perceptions – The Full Model

- Religious groups and HIV and AIDS stigma-related attitudes/perceptions were statistically significant.
- The ethnic groups as predictor variables for HIV and AIDS stigma-related attitudes were not statistically significant. For instance, being an African, Indian, mixed-race, Amerindian, Chinese or Portuguese student did not impact significantly the odds of students having inappropriate attitudes/perceptions of HIV, AIDS and PLHIV.

Relationship between HIV and AIDS Knowledge and Stigma-related Attitudes/Perceptions – The Subsets

- "HIV is not transmitted by sneezing, etc." (HIV knowledge) was significantly associated with "HIV and AIDS is death" (HIV and AIDS stigma-related perception).
- "Testing HIV-positive does not signify the contraction of AIDS" (HIV and AIDS knowledge) was significantly associated with "HIV and AIDS is not a crime" (HIV and AIDS stigma-related perception).
- "HIV infection can be contracted from insects and animals" (HIV knowledge) was significantly associated with "Uneasiness to share toilet facilities with PLHIV" (HIV and AIDS stigma-related perception).

HIV and AIDS Knowledge in Guyana

Guyanese high school students revealed moderate knowledge of HIV and AIDS, scoring correctly on an average of 7.47 out of ten items. Of the students surveyed, 97.4% recognized the modes of HIV transmission; 94.2% recognized the symptoms of HIV and AIDS; nearly half of them indicated that a blood donor is at risk of contracting HIV; and about one-fifth of the students held myths and misconceptions about HIV, AIDS and PLHIV.

The Guyana finding has some resonance with the literature. A US study (Anderson et al. 1990) showed that high school students were familiar with the two main modes of transmission – sexual intercourse and intravenous drug use – and that those with prior exposure to HIV and AIDS education had better knowledge than those without such education. Additionally, those who knew about the modes of transmission were less likely to indicate that they had two or more sexual partners. Another American study (Hancock et al. 1999) found that freshman and senior high school students had misconceptions about the modes of HIV transmission, prevention intervention and blood donation. A study of South Korean high school students (Yoo et al. 2005) showed that these students have moderate HIV and AIDS knowledge, and nearly all of them expressed the need for HIV and AIDS prevention education. Approximately half of these students expressed little concern about their susceptibility toward contracting HIV. UNAIDS (2009) reported that, apart from Thailand, all countries in Asia have an adult HIV prevalence of less than 1%. Clearly, South Korea's low HIV prevalence may account for its students' minimal interest in HIV.

A majority of Guyanese students (97.4%) indicated that HIV transmission happens (1) through unprotected sexual intercourse (vaginal, anal or oral) with HIV-infected persons, and (2) through the use of HIV contaminated needles. This finding is in sync with Tavoosi et al.'s finding (2004) that Iranian adolescents possessed knowledge about vaginal sex as an HIV transmission mode, and Odu et al.'s finding (2008) that most students at a tertiary institution were aware that using contaminated needles could transmit the infection.

However, Guyanese high school students revealed apprehension about the possibility of a blood donor contracting the infection. Similarly, Mahat and Scoloveno (2006) found that Nepalese adolescents showed minimal knowledge about HIV transmission through blood and blood testing. Guyanese high school students' fear of contagion might also be due to their misconceptions of HIV contraction, a similar mode of thinking among Portuguese adolescents (Currie et al. 2001), black and Latino high school students in San Francisco (DiClemente et al. 1988), Iranian adolescents (Yazdi et al. 2006), Iranian high school students (Tavoosi et al. 2004) and freshman and senior students from Central California (Hancock et al. 1999). The study of students in Karnataka, India (Agrawal et al. 1999), found that those with limited HIV knowledge (16.9%) were more likely to accept the myths and misconceptions of HIV transmission and prevention.

Despite having misconceptions of HIV transmission and prevention, Guyanese high school students revealed moderate HIV knowledge. This finding clearly indicates that knowledge does not comprehensively impact behaviour change. Moreover, notwithstanding Guyanese high school students' moderate knowledge of HIV, many of them still harboured misconceptions and myths about this virus. These students also revealed stigma-related attitudes/perceptions of HIV, AIDS and PLHIV. Many studies (Meng et al. 2010) found this to be the case.

Interestingly, Guyanese high school students demonstrated moderate HIV and AIDS knowledge, despite the fact that there was no formal HIV and AIDS curriculum in high schools. Compare this finding with Walker's study (1992) where New Jersey ninth graders who had no HIV and AIDS education in schools obtained a low score on the knowledge test. Imperato (1996) found that students in New York City with low knowledge of HIV carried negative attitudes about the virus. About 40% of high school students in Guyana displayed inappropriate attitudes/perceptions of HIV, AIDS and PLHIV, in spite of the finding that these students had moderate knowledge of HIV and AIDS. It would appear, therefore, that there is another variable in Guyana that may explain the moderate level of HIV and AIDS knowledge among the country's high school students; a variable that, perhaps, has more impact on attitude and behaviour than the "HIV and AIDS education in school" variable in New Jersey and elsewhere.

In Nicaragua (Manji, Pena and Dubrow 2007), adolescents with good HIV knowledge pertaining to the modes of HIV transmission expressed the view that they would care for HIV-infected persons, implying little or no fear of contagion and/or non-acceptance of misconceptions and myths of HIV prevention and transmission. The study conducted by Manji, Pena and Dubrow (2007) also indicated that stigma was high only in some areas, particularly adolescents' disapproval of sexual behaviours between people of the same gender. Yet, this Guyana study and the aforementioned studies in Portugal, San Francisco, Iran, Central California and Karnataka signified that adolescents had good to moderate knowledge of HIV and AIDS, but harboured fears of contagion and embraced misconceptions and myths about HIV, AIDS and PLHIV. With the exception of the Nicaraguan study, most of these studies suggested that education vis-à-vis knowledge of HIV and AIDS was ineffective in dismissing misconceptions and myths about HIV and AIDS, indicating the ambiguous role of education on behaviour change.

All the studies, except one (Mahat and Scoloveno 2006) in the literature review, showed that high school students recognized the modes of HIV transmission; the one exception was a study carried out among adolescents in Nepal. While Nepalese adolescents had inadequate knowledge of HIV modes of transmission, they understood that touching hands, utilizing public toilets and being bitten by mosquitoes cannot transmit the HIV infection. In addition, Nepalese adolescents rejected casual physical contact as a mode of HIV transmission, notwithstanding their inadequate knowledge of HIV. This is in contrast to Guyanese high school students with moderate knowledge of HIV, who seemed to have a concern with the potency of casual physical contact as a conduit for HIV transmission. Dias, Matos and Alves (2006) found that few Portuguese adolescents were aware that a glass, fork or spoon cannot transmit HIV; however, most Guyanese high school students knew that eating utensils would not transmit the HIV infection. Both the Guyana and Nepal studies debunked the view that HIV and AIDS knowledge may reduce risky behaviours. There must be other factors, then, in these environments which impinge on the value of knowledge in minimizing risk behaviours. Misconceptions and myths are breeding grounds for stigma and for projecting mixed messages; and with education as an active tool, a proactive review of strategies and interventions to prevent HIV and AIDS stigma-related attitudes and behaviours becomes an urgent agenda item.

Religious Groups and HIV and AIDS Knowledge

The Guyana study, through bivariate analyses, found statistical significance (p < 0.05) in median HIV and AIDS knowledge for high school students from different religious groups, indicating differences in their average scores for correct knowledge. Overall, the Guyana high school students from different religious groups – Christians (75.2%), Hindus (34%), Muslims (59.5%) and Other (71.2%) – exhibited differences on these seven knowledge areas:

- Christians understood that AIDS is a disease that weakens the human immune system.
- Hindus expressed scepticism with the scientifically accepted transmission modes vis-à-vis their concern that HIV may be spread by casual physical contact with HIV-infected persons.
- Other religious groupings of high school students (no affiliation with Christianity, Hinduism and Islam) understood that if a person tests HIV-positive, it does not follow that that person has AIDS.
- The Other groups believed there is no danger that a blood donor could contract HIV while donating blood.
- Hindus had concerns that a person could contract HIV from animals at home and from mosquitoes.
- The Hindu group expressed concerns that a person could contract HIV by being with an infected person.
- Christians believed it may be necessary to effect preventive measures for protection against contracting HIV.

On the items where students with different religious affiliations displayed differences, Guyanese students with Christian affiliation showed fewer proclivities toward assimilating and internalizing misconceptions and myths about HIV, AIDS and PLHIV. This finding has similarity with a study in Central Mozambique (Noden, Gomes and Ferreira 2010), which found that religious affiliation, in this case Christian affiliation, enhanced HIV transmission and prevention knowledge. What explains the Guyana Christian students' relative dismissal of misconceptions and myths about HIV and AIDS? Is it influenced by their religious affiliation, or is it influenced by the education that emanates from their faith-based institutions? And is there a difference between faith-based education and public education in Guyana, with respect to addressing HIV issues among their young people?

In Guyana, faith-based institutions, among others, are significant socialization agencies that shape human attitudes and behaviour; they can also be vital agents in decreasing HIV infection rates. Some faith-based institutions in Guyana are already at the forefront helping PLHIV. Nevertheless, there may be some religious institutions experiencing uneasiness in balancing their moral and spiritual concerns with the issues pertinent to HIV; such uneasiness reduces the faith-based institutions' capacity to address HIV concerns and lead HIV prevention activities within their communities.

One American Christian pastor, Reverend Danyiel Griffin, of El Bethel Baptist Church, Flint, Michigan, expressed his concerns, thus: "We hear you. We know that HIV is a serious health problem. As a church, what we don't know is how to bridge the gap between what the church sees as its moral responsibility and the current HIV messages of condom use. It goes against everything that the church stands for."

It is clear that in the Guyana finding, some faith-based groups may need to build capacity to address HIV concerns. One example is where YBH (Your Blessed Health) was utilized to build capacity (Griffith et al. 2010). The YBH HIV-prevention efforts were effective through adherence to these principles: "(1) respect the denominational doctrines and visions of the pastors, (2) engage pastors' spouses (or some other group as champions), and (3) build on the church leadership teams' understanding of what is appropriate and will be acceptable in their specific organizations" (Griffith et al. 2010). Another study (Francis et al. 2009) examined African American faith-based leaders' beliefs and attitudes in offering HIV prevention education and services to adolescents. They found that leaders expressed a keenness to deliver abstinence messages, and that they would address concerns pertaining to health education, but would not speak of issues relating to HIV.

Lindley et al. (2010) conducted a study of African American parishioners from Project FAITH (Fostering AIDS Initiatives that Heal) churches in South Carolina. They found that parishioners showed good HIV knowledge on modes of transmission through unprotected sexual intercourse and the use of contaminated needles, but harboured misconceptions, believing that transmission of HIV may occur through casual contact, mosquito bites, blood donation and HIV testing. Students from different religious groups in Guyana, like the Christians in Project FAITH churches, recognized that HIV transmission happens through unprotected sex and using contaminated needles; however, inconsistency exists between the Guyana Christian students who displayed less receptiveness to myths and misconceptions and the Project FAITH Christian parishioners who had little understanding of these misapprehensions. However, Project FAITH parishioners' feelings toward misconceptions and myths of HIV transmission were similar to those of the Guyana Hindu and Other (non-Christian, non-Hindu and non-Muslim) students. There is also another similarity where both Other Guyana students and Project FAITH parishioners exhibited poor knowledge of HIV transmission through blood donation.

The answer to Guyana Christian students' relative dismissal of misconceptions and myths about HIV and AIDS may be found in a Malawi study (Trinitapoli 2009). This study found that persons from Christian congregations, where clergy often delivered formal HIV messages, supervised the sexual behaviours of its congregation and surreptitiously promoted condom use, showed better adherence to the ABCs of HIV prevention. Assuming that the Guyana Christian students were ardent church goers, then their places of worship may have the answer to their relative dismissal of the myths and misconceptions about HIV. Jamaican adolescents who were devoted to the church tended to possess good HIV and AIDS knowledge (Robillard 2001). Could it be that the Guyana Christian students are committed to the teachings of the church and that facilitated their relative dismissal of myths and misconceptions about HIV and AIDS? Or is there another explanation?

HIV and AIDS Stigma-related Attitudes/ Perceptions in Guyana

There is a general feeling in Guyana that HIV and AIDS has an association with homosexuals and women sex workers. This perpetual mindset persists, having its genesis in 1987, when a male homosexual was identified and diagnosed as the first HIV case in Guyana. This sustained mindset remains a fertile breeding ground for sexual prejudices. In Guyana, therefore, it is not surprising that only a small proportion of male (58.4%) and female (60.6%) high school students displayed appropriate attitudes/ perceptions of HIV, AIDS and PLHIV. About two-thirds of Christian and Muslim students projected an appropriate outlook toward HIV, AIDS and PLHIV. About two-thirds of African and Amerindian students showed appropriate attitudes/perceptions of HIV, AIDS and PLHIV. A small proportion of both the 13–15 (59.5%) and 16–18 (59.8%) age groups had appropriate attitudes/perceptions of HIV, AIDS and PLHIV.

Clearly, HIV and AIDS stigma-related attitudes are a complex phenomenon among a sample of high school students in Guyana. Overall, only 60% of high school students showed appropriate attitudes/perceptions and 40% showed inappropriate attitudes/perceptions. Students revealed inappropriate attitudes/perceptions in spite of their moderate knowledge of HIV and AIDS.

Similarly, Kenyan high school students with correspondingly adequate HIV and AIDS knowledge still engaged in negative behaviours (Pattullo et al. 1994), in other words, they engaged in high-risk sexual behaviours and did not use condoms. There are those studies that found limited HIV and AIDS knowledge was associated with negative attitudes toward PLHIV. For instance most Iranian high school students with inadequate HIV knowledge, displayed these stigma-related attitudes: HIV testing should become mandatory before marriage, people who are HIV-positive should face quarantine and HIV is a sin (Yazdi et al. 2006).

Adolescents in Nepal (Mahat and Scoloveno 2006) saw AIDS as an immense problem, and had apprehensions toward HIV, AIDS and PLHIV. Adolescents in Nigeria (Odusanya and Bankole 2006) also carried a negative mindset; they were not willing to eat on a clean plate or drink from a cup that was used by an HIV-infected person. They took the view that schools should not admit HIV-infected students, PLHIV should not be allowed to work and they generally ended relationships with PLHIV. Adolescents in Portugal also expressed negative views about PLHIV (Dias, Matos and Alves 2006) just as much as the Guyana high school students. The Portuguese construed that AIDS was incurable and believed that poor HIV and AIDS knowledge induced discrimination against PLHIV.

The Guyana findings revealed some deep-seated negative attitudes/perceptions toward PLHIV, and are consistent with Norman, Carr and Jimenez's study in Jamaica (2006). The Jamaican study was intended to determine the attitudes of university students toward PLHIV. These students showed less sympathy toward PLHIV, especially male homosexuals or women sex workers, but they garnered some sympathy for heterosexual PLHIV and women (non-sex workers) living with HIV. Previous studies showed that negative attitudes may have links with sexual prejudices. Breault and Polifroni (1992) conducted a qualitative study to identify the attitudes and feelings of nurses caring for PLHIV. They found six themes that characterized the nurses' feelings and attitudes: fear, anger, sympathy, self-enhancement, fatigue and helplessness. These nurses engendered negative perceptions and treatments for AIDS patients who were drug users and homosexuals. It would appear, then, that sexual prejudices and the fear of AIDS as a terminal disease among these nurses could have triggered stigma-related attitudes.

Multiple Logistic Regression Analysis

In the multiple logistic regression analysis, gender as the predictor variable for both HIV and AIDS knowledge and stigma-related attitudes was dropped, as the bivariate analysis showed no statistical significance, and age was identified as a confounder for HIV and AIDS stigma-related attitudes.

Bivariate analyses in this study indicated that there was statistical significance in the median scores for HIV and AIDS stigma-related attitudes among the religious groups, and the different religious groups had different scores for HIV and AIDS stigma-related attitudes. The logistic regression analyses showed that religious groups were significant predictors of HIV and AIDS stigma-related attitudes. This finding is not surprising, as the most important blockade against African American faith-based organizations presenting a potent answer to HIV and AIDS is the damaging moral and religious attitudes and behaviours on HIV transmission (Francis and Liverpool 2009).

Implications

Undoubtedly, limited understanding of the myths and misconceptions of HIV and AIDS indicates that prevention education and awareness policy must focus more than ever on how HIV is not transmitted. Those who stigmatize PLHIV perceive them as shamefully different, and generally dole out a label, not only to the behaviour, but also to the person. The label becomes a stigma, a mark of social disgrace that separates PLHIV from those who see themselves as "normal". Thus, myths and misconceptions drive stigmatizing behaviours toward HIV, AIDS and PLHIV.

In this study, Hindu students and those from Other religious groups (excluding Christians and Muslims) show greater proclivity than Christian students to accept misconceptions and myths about HIV and AIDS. The Guyana Ministry of Health study showed that both in-school and out-of-school young people have misconceptions and myths about HIV and AIDS (Ministry of Health, 2008), producing some consistency with this study. This finding may have resonance with a Trinidad & Tobago study (Genrich and Braithwaite 2005) which defined the Hindu representative's position as uneasy in addressing HIV and AIDS. This uneasiness came not only from Hindus, but also from other faith-based quarters: the Open Bible, Unity of Women, Seventh Day Adventist and Jamaat al Muslimeen.

Given that heterosexual transmission is the main mode of spreading HIV infection, it is appropriate to conclude that high risk sexual behaviours are prevalent and are the drivers of the epidemic in Guyana. With heterosexual transmission accounting for more than 90% of seropositive cases, we should know whether persons engaging in risky behaviours want to change such behaviours in order to reduce the probability of contracting the HIV infection.

However, the literature review in this book is in synchrony with the findings of the Guyana study, which show that, notwithstanding good to moderate HIV and AIDS knowledge among high school students, these students still produced behaviours that harboured myths and misconceptions about HIV and AIDS. It also showed that students with good to moderate knowledge displayed orientations toward risky behaviours and stigma-related attitudes toward PLHIV, HIV and AIDS. What is the explanation for such behaviours?

The answer to this question in Ajzen's theory of planned behaviour is "irrationality". Using Ajzen's language, the Guyana high school students' attitudes, their subjective norms and their perceptions of behavioural control did not stem from their behavioural, normative and control beliefs. In fact, in a state of irrationality, the student's intentions were not yet formed to effect desired behaviours. Azjen's theory of planned behaviour suggests that the individual person is rational, and so would process information first, in order to form intentions to produce desired behaviours. This line of thinking indicates that Ajzen's model does incorporate a theory of action by virtue of a person's capacity to form intentions; that is, people are knowledgeable and capable of reflexively monitoring their behaviours and are aware of the conditions governing their behaviours (Giddens 1979). For these reasons, given that the Guyana students' moderate knowledge led to stigmatized attitudes of HIV, AIDS and PLHIV, the theory of planned behaviour would consider such behaviours as unplanned or irrational because those students' intentions were not yet created and there was inadequate perceived behavioural control (self-efficacy), and hence, they were ill prepared to engage in any desired behaviours. Azjen (2011) would argue that without intentions, a person would be in a state of uneasiness to activate a rational behaviour. Nonetheless, these students do have the knowledge and capability to form intentions and to engage in rational behaviours.

Again, following Azjen, once a person's intentions are constituted, the person is in a state of readiness to activate reduced risk behaviours and negative attitudes toward PLHIV, HIV and AIDS. For this reason, too, inadequate or absent intentions producing a state of irrationality among the Guyana high school students could induce them to embrace myths and misconceptions of HIV and AIDS, and rational thinking possibly emerges with the presence of intention. Rational choice theory explains these students' possible inclination toward reduced risky behaviours and reduced negativity toward PLHIV, HIV and AIDS, thus: where these students assess the cost/benefit scenario of a situation and then decide that they will choose the option with the greatest benefits at the least cost and we can use Becker et al.'s *Health Belief Model* (1977) to apply the principles of rational choice theory. Under the *Health Belief Model*, these students may act to protect themselves if they see themselves as susceptible to a health problem, if they see that problem as serious and if the benefits of taking protective actions offset the costs of taking those actions. However, rational choice behaviour, in the first place, would require the students to have an intention and self-efficacy; that is, students should have the motivation and ability to reduce stigma-related attitudes toward HIV, AIDS and PLHIV.

Without intentions and self-efficacy, HIV and AIDS knowledge would have minimal impact and relevance on reducing stigma-related attitudes and perceptions.

This study bears several limitations. (1) The study used convenience sampling, a non-probability sampling where teachers selected students on the basis of availability, biasing sample representativeness, which makes it difficult to determine the level of outcome (dependent variable) emanating from cause (independent variable). (2) Being a cross-sectional design limits the study's capacity to make a case for causation. (3) One high school with strong religious doctrine and largely from one religious group provided the total sample with 61 (78%) students from its Grades 10 and 11 student population. The other high schools together presented an average of 11% from their Grades 10 and 11 toward the total sample. It is possible that this religious school's students would skew the findings of students from the same religious group who attended other schools.

Recommendations for a future research agenda to show public health significance, that is, whether improved HIV and AIDS knowledge produces positive attitudes and perceptions of HIV and AIDS and people living with HIV and AIDS, may include these areas: develop common measurement tools with internal and external validation for HIV and AIDS knowledge and stigma-related attitudes and perceptions, as the existing measurement tools are inadequate and dissimilar; design a knowledge instrument on the basis of formative research concentrating on HIV and AIDS concerns aimed at a specific target population, and then apply the formative data to develop knowledge components to target negative attitudes and perceptions of HIV and AIDS and people living with HIV and AIDS; study health outcomes possibly arising from improved knowledge and positive attitudes and perceptions, in order to establish their potency for universal applications; and focus on the non-normative knowledge aspects, that is, myths and misconceptions, since they are the only predictors of negative attitudes and perceptions of HIV and AIDS and people living with HIV and AIDS in this study. At this juncture, HIV and AIDS knowledge and education may effect positive behavioural change in stigma-related attitudes and perceptions, but the precondition for this change is that people must have intentions and self-efficacy. Myths and misconceptions predominate without intention and self-efficacy.

Gender and HIV
and AIDS Knowledge

Variables/Question	Correct n (%)			Not Correct n (%)		
	Male n (%)	Female n (%)	Total N (%)	Male n (%)	Female n (%)	Total N (%)
1. AIDS is a disease that weakens the human body's immune system, making it difficult to fight infections and exposing persons infected to a number of serious, often fatal illnesses (**True**).	151 (94)	199 (91.3)	350 (92.3)	10 (6)	19 (8.7)	29 (7.7)
2. Loss of appetite, weight loss, fever, night sweats, skin rashes, diarrhoea, tiredness, lack of resistance to infection or swollen lymph nodes are signs and symptoms of AIDS or other AIDS-related conditions (**True**).	147 (91.3)	210 (96.3)	357 (94.2)	14 (8.7)	8 (3.7)	22 (5.8)
3. HIV is spread by casual physical contact with people who are infected – such as hugging, handshaking, travelling in the same vehicle, touching the same papers, or sharing the same office furniture, telephone or computer (**False**).	143 (88.8)	174 (79.8)	317 (83.6)	18 (11.2)	44 (20.2)	62 (16.4)
4. HIV is spread through unprotected sexual intercourse, vaginally, anally or orally, with infected persons; use of or sharing contaminated needles with infected persons; mother-to-child transmissions during pregnancy or childbirth; and sometimes through transfusions or other exchanges of HIV-infected blood (**True**).	174 (79.8)	185 (84.9)	308 (80.6)	44 (20.2)	33 (15.1)	71 (19.4)
5. HIV can be transmitted by sneezing, coughing, using sinks, bathrooms, toilets, the same eating or drinking utensils, or eating food prepared by an infected person (**False**).	123 (76.4)	185 (84.9)	308 (80.6)	38 (23.6)	33 (15.1)	71 (19.4)

	Correct n (%)			Not Correct n (%)		
Variables/Question	**Male n (%)**	**Female n (%)**	**Total N (%)**	**Male n (%)**	**Female n (%)**	**Total N (%)**
6. If a person tests positive for HIV when they take the antibody test, it does not mean that they have AIDS. In fact, a person who has HIV may show no signs or symptoms of the disease and may not develop AIDS for many years *(True)*.	134 (83.2)	181 (83)	315 (83.1)	27 (16.8)	37 (17)	64 (16.9)
7. There is no danger at all that a blood donor could get HIV while giving blood *(True)*.	95 (59)	117 (53.7)	167 (44.1)	66 (41)	101 (46.3)	212 (55.9)
8. A person can get HIV from animals around the home such as cats and dogs and from mosquitoes *(False)*.	132 (82)	175 (80.3)	307 (81)	29 (18)	43 (19.7)	72 (19)
9. A person is likely to contract HIV by being or working around someone who is infected on a daily basis over a long period of time *(False)*.	143 (88.8)	173 (79.4)	316 (83.4)	18 (11.2)	45 (20.6)	63 (16.6)
10. To protect yourself and/or those you work with from being infected with HIV, you will need to take or put into place preventative measures *(True)*.	110 (68.3)	155 (71.1)	265 (70)	51 (31.7)	63 (28.9)	114 (30)

Age and HIV and AIDS Knowledge

		Casual physical contact		
		False	**True**	**Total**
Age 13–15	Count	112	36	148
	% within Age	75.7%	24.3%	100.0%
	% within casual physical contact	35.3%	58.1%	39.1%
Age 16–18	Count	203	26	229
	% within Age	88.6%	11.4%	100.0%
	% within casual physical contact	64.0%	41.9%	60.4%

Age * Human animal transmission cross-tabulation

		Human animal transmission		Total
		.00	1.00	
Age 13–15	Count	106	42	148
	% within Age	71.6%	28.4%	100.0%
	% within human animal transmission	34.5%	58.3%	39.1%
Age 16–18	Count	199	30	229
	% within Age	86.9%	13.1%	100.0%
	% within human animal transmission	64.8%	41.7%	60.4%

Age * Working with HIV-infected persons cross-tabulation

		Working with HIV-infected persons		Total
		.00	1.00	
Age 13–15	Count	113	35	148
	% within Age	76.4%	23.6%	100.0%
	% within working with HIV-infected persons	35.8%	55.6%	39.1%
Age 16–18	Count	201	28	229
	% within Age	87.8%	12.2%	100.0%
	% within working with HIV-infected persons	63.6%	44.4%	60.4%

One-way Analysis of Variance

Variables:
Correct Attitude ~ Religious groups = 1
Correct Attitude ~ Religious groups = 3
Correct Attitude ~ Religious groups = 4
Correct Attitude ~ Religious groups = 2

Source of Variation	Sum Squares	DF	Mean Square
Between Groups	65.666764	3	21.888921
Within Groups	1518.818724	375	4.050183
Corrected Total	1584.485488	378	

F (variance ratio) = 5.404427
P = 0.0012

ANOVA

		Sum of Squares	df	Mean Square	F	Sig.
Death	Between Groups	1.785	3	.595	2.489	.060
	Within Groups	89.640	375	.239		
	Total	91.425	378			
Punishment	Between Groups	.981	3	.327	1.308	.271
	Within Groups	93.716	375	.250		
	Total	94.697	378			

ANOVA (continued)

		Sum of Squares	df	Mean Square	F	Sig.
Crime	Between Groups	.746	3	.249	3.702	.012
	Within Groups	25.186	375	.067		
	Total	25.931	378			
Happens to others	Between Groups	.136	3	.045	1.059	.366
	Within Groups	16.101	375	.043		
	Total	16.237	378			
Horror	Between Groups	.191	3	.064	.273	.845
	Within Groups	87.561	375	.233		
	Total	87.752	378			
Jokes	Between Groups	.154	3	.051	.554	.646
	Within Groups	34.833	375	.093		
	Total	34.987	378			
Gossip	Between Groups	.030	3	.010	.181	.909
	Within Groups	20.693	375	.055		
	Total	20.723	378			
Not work	Between Groups	.154	3	.051	.745	.526
	Within Groups	25.778	375	.069		
	Total	25.931	378			
Not sell food	Between Groups	1.182	3	.394	1.735	.159
	Within Groups	85.145	375	.227		
	Total	86.327	378			

ANOVA (continued)

		Sum of Squares	df	Mean Square	F	Sig.
Not comfortable	Between Groups	.287	3	.096	.588	.623
	Within Groups	61.069	375	.163		
	Total	61.356	378			
Not sharing work tools	Between Groups	1.314	3	.438	3.487	.016
	Within Groups	47.113	375	.126		
	Total	48.427	378			
Not sharing toilet	Between Groups	3.323	3	1.108	5.356	.001
	Within Groups	77.558	375	.207		
	Total	80.881	378			
Sitting next to person	Between Groups	1.382	3	.461	1.859	.136
	Within Groups	92.887	375	.248		
	Total	94.269	378			

Games-Howell Test

Multiple Comparisons

Dependent Variable		(I) Religious groups		(J) Religious groups		Mean Difference (I–J)	Std. Error	Sig.	95% Confidence Interval Lower Bound	95% Confidence Interval Upper Bound
d1	Death	d2	Christian	d3	Hindu	-.16494*	.06024	.034	-.3212	-.0087
			Hindu	d3	Christian	.16494*	.06024	.034	.0087	.3212
					Muslim	.03274	.10878	.990	-.2529	.3184
	Crime	d2	Christian	d3	Hindu	-.10171	.03899	.050	-.2034	.0000
					Muslim	-.04643	.04729	.760	-.1729	.0801
					Other	-.08073	.04656	.316	-.2038	.0423
			Hindu	d3	Christian	.10171	.03899	.050	.0000	.2034
	Happens to others	d2	Christian	d3	Hindu	-.02858	.03032	.782	-.1075	.0503
					Muslim	.03960*	.01376	.023	.0040	.0752
					Other	-.01809	.03543	.956	-.1113	.0751
			Muslim	d3	Christian	-.03960*	.01376	.023	-.0752	-.0040
	Not sharing work tools	d2	Christian	d3	Hindu	-.14604*	.05117	.026	-.2793	-.0128
					Muslim	-.05820	.06510	.808	-.2318	.1154
					Other	-.04989	.05492	.800	-.1944	.0946
			Hindu	d3	Christian	.14604*	.05117	.026	.0128	.2793
					Muslim	.08784	.07700	.666	-.1143	.2900
					Other	.09615	.06861	.501	-.0826	.2749
	Not sharing toilet	d2	Christian	d3	Hindu	-.22480*	.06170	.002	-.3851	-.0645
					Muslim	-.04482	.08211	.947	-.2633	.1736
			Hindu	d3	Christian	.22480*	.06170	.002	.0645	.3851
					Other	.22727*	.08090	.029	.0165	.4381
			Other	d3	Hindu	-.22727*	.08090	.029	-.4381	-.0165

*The mean difference is significant at the 0.05 level.

Kruskal-Wallis (Ranks): Ethnic Groups and Attitudes/ Perceptions

	Race	N	Mean Rank
Death	African	154	172.25
	Indian	146	200.80
	Chinese	6	172.25
	Amerindian	15	178.57
	Portuguese	10	191.20
	Mixed	48	219.63
	Total	379	
Punishment	African	154	182.41
	Indian	146	197.44
	Chinese	6	223.83
	Amerindian	15	185.93
	Portuguese	10	211.20
	Mixed	48	184.35
	Total	379	

	Race	N	Mean Rank
Crime	African	154	184.61
	Indian	146	191.58
	Chinese	6	239.17
	Amerindian	15	176.00
	Portuguese	10	194.95
	Mixed	48	199.69
	Total	379	
Happens to others	African	154	190.11
	Indian	146	189.29
	Chinese	6	213.08
	Amerindian	15	194.13
	Portuguese	10	200.45
	Mixed	48	185.45
	Total	379	
Horror	African	154	188.86
	Indian	146	186.32
	Chinese	6	227.42
	Amerindian	15	183.20
	Portuguese	10	240.05
	Mixed	48	191.89
	Total	379	
Jokes	African	154	184.89
	Indian	146	190.03
	Chinese	6	209.50
	Amerindian	15	209.50
	Portuguese	10	190.55
	Mixed	48	197.66
	Total	379	

	Race	N	Mean Rank
Gossip	African	154	192.39
	Indian	146	188.02
	Chinese	6	201.00
	Amerindian	15	201.00
	Portuguese	10	182.05
	Mixed	48	185.21
	Total	379	
Not work	African	154	190.77
	Indian	146	191.58
	Chinese	6	176.00
	Amerindian	15	176.00
	Portuguese	10	194.95
	Mixed	48	187.84
	Total	379	
Not sell food	African	154	182.56
	Indian	146	194.89
	Chinese	6	218.25
	Amerindian	15	199.30
	Portuguese	10	218.25
	Mixed	48	186.67
	Total	379	
Not comfortable	African	154	187.19
	Indian	146	187.84
	Chinese	6	277.83
	Amerindian	15	189.40
	Portuguese	10	208.35
	Mixed	48	190.98
	Total	379	

	Race	N	Mean Rank
Not sharing work tools	African	154	179.96
	Indian	146	193.95
	Chinese	6	287.83
	Amerindian	15	186.77
	Portuguese	10	199.40
	Mixed	48	197.03
	Total	379	
Not sharing toilet	African	154	177.03
	Indian	146	201.59
	Chinese	6	289.42
	Amerindian	15	156.77
	Portuguese	10	226.25
	Mixed	48	186.77
	Total	379	
Sitting next to person	African	154	184.44
	Indian	146	194.15
	Chinese	6	259.92
	Amerindian	15	177.80
	Portuguese	10	234.65
	Mixed	48	180.96
	Total	379	

HIV and AIDS Knowledge – Full Model

Logistic regression

Warning: result not of full rank. There is more than one solution for the model.

Deviance goodness of fit chi-square =	13.994289	df = 25	P = 0.9618
Deviance (likelihood ratio) chi-square =	10.475933	df = 9	P = 0.3133
Intercept	b0 = –1.911767	z = –8.975735	P < 0.0001
Age	b1 = 0.072843	z = 0.484026	P = 0.6284
Religious Group (1)	b2 = –0.338755	z = –2.789538	P = 0.0053
Religious Group (2)	b3 = –0.756398	z = –4.158483	P < 0.0001
Religious Group (3)	b4 = –0.440459	z = –2.125444	P = 0.0335
Religious Group (4)	b5 = –0.376155	z = –2.232229	P = 0.0256
Ethnic Group (1)	b6 = –0.111643	z = –0.668539	P = 0.5038
Ethnic Group (2)	b7 = –0.212484	z = –1.193126	P = 0.2328
Ethnic Group (3)	b8 = –0.445555	z = –0.855964	P = 0.392
Ethnic Group (4)	b9 = –0.021273	z = –0.071061	P = 0.9433
Ethnic Group (5)	b10 = –0.662628	z = –1.459776	P = 0.1444
Ethnic Group (6)	b11 = –0.458185	z = –1.930083	P = 0.0536

logit Scale = –1.911767 +0.072843 Age –0.338755 Religious Group (1) –0.756398 Religious Group (2) –0.440459 Religious Group (3) –0.376155 Religious Group (4) –0.111643 Ethnic Group (1) –0.212484 Ethnic Group (2) –0.445555 Ethnic Group (3) –0.021273 Ethnic Group (4) –0.662628 Ethnic Group (5) –0.458185 Ethnic Group (6)

Logistic regression – odds ratios

Parameter	Estimate	Odds Ratio	95% CI
Constant	−1.911767		
Age	0.072843	1.075562	0.800819 to 1.444563
Religious Group (1)	−0.338755	0.712657	0.561711 to 0.904167
Religious Group (2)	−0.756398	0.469354	0.328604 to 0.670391
Religious Group (3)	−0.440459	0.643741	0.42886 to 0.966289
Religious Group (4)	−0.376155	0.686496	0.493402 to 0.955157
Ethnic Group (1)	−0.111643	0.894363	0.644714 to 1.240684
Ethnic Group (2)	−0.212484	0.808573	0.570334 to 1.146331
Ethnic Group (3)	−0.445555	0.640469	0.230899 to 1.776536
Ethnic Group (4)	−0.021273	0.978952	0.544436 to 1.760256
Ethnic Group (5)	−0.662628	0.515495	0.21176 to 1.25489
Ethnic Group (6)	−0.458185	0.632431	0.397142 to 1.007119

The Ten HIV and AIDS Knowledge Items

Logistic regression

Warning: result not of full rank, there is more than one solution for the model.

Deviance goodness of fit chi-square =	2.086713	df = 25	P > 0.9999
Deviance (likelihood ratio) chi-square =	0.561691	df = 9	P > 0.9999
Intercept	b0 = −1.343025	z = −7.933147	P < 0.0001
Age	b1 = −0.017883	z = −0.144113	P = 0.8854
Religion (1)	b2 = −0.331476	z = −3.323726	P = 0.0009
Religion (2)	b3 = −0.345284	z = −2.598501	P = 0.0094
Religion (3)	b4 = −0.355555	z = −2.084931	P = 0.0371
Religion (4)	b5 = −0.31071	z = −2.19553	P = 0.0281
Ethnic Groups (1)	b6 = −0.297557	z = −2.228964	P = 0.0258
Ethnic Groups (2)	b7 = −0.214704	z = −1.563135	P = 0.118
Ethnic Groups (3)	b8 = −0.146462	z = −0.382469	P = 0.7021
Ethnic Groups (4)	b9 = −0.282647	z = −1.055026	P = 0.2914
Ethnic Groups (5)	b10 = −0.165344	z = −0.544132	P = 0.5864
Ethnic Groups (6)	b11 = −0.23631	z = −1.340588	P = 0.1801

logit Ques1 = −1.343025 −0.017883 Age −0.331476 Religion (1) −0.345284 Religion (2) − 0.355555 Religion (3) −0.31071 Religion (4) −0.297557 Ethnic Groups (1) −0.214704 Ethnic Groups (2) −0.146462 Ethnic Groups (3) −0.282647 Ethnic Groups (4) −0.165344 Ethnic Groups (5) −0.23631 Ethnic Groups (6)

Logistic regression – odds ratios

Parameter	Estimate	Odds Ratio	95% CI
Constant	–1.343025		
Age	–0.017883	0.982276	0.770207 to 1.252736
Religion (1)	–0.331476	0.717864	0.590407 to 0.872836
Religion (2)	–0.345284	0.70802	0.545682 to 0.918652
Religion (3)	–0.355555	0.700784	0.501677 to 0.978914
Religion (4)	–0.31071	0.732926	0.555391 to 0.967212
Ethnic Groups (1)	–0.297557	0.74263	0.571664 to 0.964727
Ethnic Groups (2)	–0.214704	0.80678	0.616366 to 1.056019
Ethnic Groups (3)	–0.146462	0.863758	0.407788 to 1.829574
Ethnic Groups (4)	–0.282647	0.753786	0.445868 to 1.274352
Ethnic Groups (5)	–0.165344	0.847602	0.467238 to 1.537607
Ethnic Groups (6)	–0.23631	0.789536	0.558892 to 1.115362

Logistic regression

Warning: rank changed, consider dropping predictors.
Warning: result not of full rank, there is more than one solution for the model.

Deviance goodness of fit chi-square =	3.603058	df = 25	P > 0.9999
Deviance (likelihood ratio) chi-square =	7.294919	df = 9	P = 0.6064
Intercept	$b0 = -1.296859$	$z = -7.736445$	P < 0.0001
Age	$b1 = -0.029555$	$z = -0.240675$	P = 0.8098
Religion (1)	$b2 = -0.472611$	$z = -4.697506$	P < 0.0001
Religion (2)	$b3 = -0.097855$	$z = -0.77253$	P = 0.4398
Religion (3)	$b4 = -0.361928$	$z = -2.13365$	P = 0.0329
Religion (4)	$b5 = -0.364466$	$z = -2.575891$	P = 0.01
Ethnic Groups (1)	$b6 = -0.210136$	$z = -1.545451$	P = 0.1222
Ethnic Groups (2)	$b7 = -0.272553$	$z = -1.949276$	P = 0.0513
Ethnic Groups (3)	$b8 = -0.086805$	$z = -0.226212$	P = 0.821
Ethnic Groups (4)	$b9 = -0.394195$	$z = -1.388787$	P = 0.1649
Ethnic Groups (5)	$b10 = -0.267346$	$z = -0.842821$	P = 0.3993
Ethnic Groups (6)	$b11 = -0.065824$	$z = -0.385224$	P = 0.7001

logit Ques2 = –1.296859 –0.029555 Age –0.472611 Religion (1) –0.097855 Religion (2) – 0.361928 Religion (3) –0.364466 Religion (4) –0.210136 Ethnic Groups (1) –0.272553 Ethnic Groups (2) –0.086805 Ethnic Groups (3) –0.394195 Ethnic Groups (4) –0.267346 Ethnic Groups (5) –0.065824 Ethnic Groups (6)

Logistic regression - odds ratios

Parameter	Estimate	Odds Ratio	95% CI
Constant	−1.296859		
Age	−0.029555	0.970878	0.763199 to 1.235069
Religion (1)	−0.472611	0.623373	0.511811 to 0.759253
Religion (2)	−0.097855	0.90678	0.707427 to 1.162311
Religion (3)	−0.361928	0.696332	0.499377 to 0.970968
Religion (4)	−0.364466	0.694568	0.526353 to 0.916541
Ethnic Groups (1)	−0.210136	0.810474	0.62087 to 1.05798
Ethnic Groups (2)	−0.272553	0.761433	0.578914 to 1.001496
Ethnic Groups (3)	−0.086805	0.916856	0.432182 to 1.945072
Ethnic Groups (4)	−0.394195	0.674222	0.386542 to 1.176006
Ethnic Groups (5)	−0.267346	0.765408	0.411045 to 1.425271
Ethnic Groups (6)	−0.065824	0.936296	0.669833 to 1.308759

Logistic regression

Warning: result not of full rank, there is more than one solution for the model.

Deviance goodness of fit chi-square =	25.839242	df = 25	P = 0.4162
Deviance (likelihood ratio) chi-square =	116.91032	df = 9	P < 0.0001
Intercept	$b0 = -5.957934$	z = −0.018706	P = 0.9851
Age	$b1 = -0.402583$	z = −1.419801	P = 0.1557
Religion (1)	$b2 = -2.767223$	z = −0.034753	P = 0.9723
Religion (2)	$b3 = -0.455384$	z = −0.005719	P = 0.9954
Religion (3)	$b4 = -1.839262$	z = −0.023098	P = 0.9816
Religion (4)	$b5 = -0.896065$	z = −0.011253	P = 0.991
Ethnic Groups (1)	$b6 = 2.741475$	z = 0.006886	P = 0.9945
Ethnic Groups (2)	$b7 = 4.339387$	z = 0.010899	P = 0.9913
Ethnic Groups (3)	$b8 = 4.494858$	z = 0.01129	P = 0.991
Ethnic Groups (4)	$b9 = -11.700427$	z = −0.006918	P = 0.9945
Ethnic Groups (5)	$b10 = -11.221899$	z = −0.006919	P = 0.9945
Ethnic Groups (6)	$b11 = 5.388673$	z = 0.013535	P = 0.9892

logit Ques3 = −5.957934 −0.402583 Age −2.767223 Religion (1) −0.455384 Religion (2) − 1.839262 Religion (3) −0.896065 Religion (4) +2.741475 Ethnic Groups (1) +4.339387 Ethnic Groups (2) +4.494858 Ethnic Groups (3) −11.700427 Ethnic Groups (4) −11.221899 Ethnic Groups (5) +5.388673 Ethnic Groups (6)

Logistic regression – odds ratios

Parameter	Estimate	Odds Ratio	95% CI
Constant	–5.957934		
Age	–0.402583	0.668591	0.383533 to 1.165514
Religion (1)	–2.767223	0.062836	1.05E-69 to 3.77074209412823E+66
Religion (2)	–0.455384	0.634204	1.06E-68 to 3.80274101279476E+67
Religion (3)	–1.839262	0.158935	2.65E-69 to 9.5482180244646E+66
Religion (4)	–0.896065	0.408172	6.80E-69 to 2.44862782213953E+67
Ethnic Groups (1)	2.741475	15.509838	* to *
Ethnic Groups (2)	4.339387	76.66055	* to *
Ethnic Groups (3)	4.494858	89.555422	* to *
Ethnic Groups (4)	–11.700427	0.000008	* to *
Ethnic Groups (5)	–11.221899	0.000013	* to *
Ethnic Groups (6)	5.388673	218.912637	* to *

Logistic regression

Warning: result not of full rank, there is more than one solution for the model.

Deviance goodness of fit chi-square =	3.428073	df = 25	P > 0.9999
Deviance (likelihood ratio) chi-square =	7.83203	df = 9	P = 0.5512
Intercept	$b0 = -1.264849$	$z = -7.662655$	P < 0.0001
Age	$b1 = -0.024572$	$z = -0.202837$	P = 0.8393
Religion (1)	$b2 = -0.425236$	$z = -4.294526$	P < 0.0001
Religion (2)	$b3 = -0.071335$	$z = -0.572557$	P = 0.5669
Religion (3)	$b4 = -0.361053$	$z = -2.15467$	P = 0.0312
Religion (4)	$b5 = -0.407226$	$z = -2.871391$	P = 0.0041
Ethnic Groups (1)	$b6 = -0.275191$	$z = -2.061818$	P = 0.0392
Ethnic Groups (2)	$b7 = -0.28128$	$z = -2.056553$	P = 0.0397
Ethnic Groups (3)	$b8 = -0.135876$	$z = -0.354825$	P = 0.7227
Ethnic Groups (4)	$b9 = -0.264465$	$z = -0.988128$	P = 0.3231
Ethnic Groups (5)	$b10 = -0.22406$	$z = -0.737402$	P = 0.4609
Ethnic Groups (6)	$b11 = -0.083977$	$z = -0.501909$	P = 0.6157

logit Ques4 = –1.264849 –0.024572 Age –0.425236 Religion (1) –0.071335 Religion (2) – 0.361053 Religion (3) –0.407226 Religion (4) –0.275191 Ethnic Groups (1) –0.28128 Ethnic Groups (2) –0.135876 Ethnic Groups (3) –0.264465 Ethnic Groups (4) –0.22406 Ethnic Groups (5) –0.083977 Ethnic Groups (6)

Logistic regression – odds ratios

Parameter	Estimate	Odds Ratio	95% CI
Constant	–1.264849		
Age	–0.024572	0.975727	0.769507 to 1.237212
Religion (1)	–0.425236	0.653616	0.538317 to 0.793609
Religion (2)	–0.071335	0.93115	0.729404 to 1.188697
Religion (3)	–0.361053	0.696942	0.501838 to 0.9679
Religion (4)	–0.407226	0.665494	0.503994 to 0.878745
Ethnic Groups (1)	–0.275191	0.759427	0.584623 to 0.986497
Ethnic Groups (2)	–0.28128	0.754817	0.577325 to 0.986876
Ethnic Groups (3)	–0.135876	0.872951	0.412129 to 1.849043
Ethnic Groups (4)	–0.264465	0.767617	0.454284 to 1.297065
Ethnic Groups (5)	–0.22406	0.799268	0.44061 to 1.449873
Ethnic Groups (6)	–0.083977	0.919452	0.662384 to 1.276287

Logistic regression

Warning: result not of full rank, there is more than one solution for the model.

Deviance goodness of fit chi-square =	9.242283	df = 25	P = 0.9982
Deviance (likelihood ratio) chi-square =	7.121896	df = 9	P = 0.6244
Intercept	b0 = –1.370984	z = –7.762147	P < 0.0001
Age	b1 = –0.026447	z = –0.201844	P = 0.84
Religion (1)	b2 = –0.411853	z = –3.851038	P = 0.0001
Religion (2)	b3 = –0.089442	z = –0.659227	P = 0.5098
Religion (3)	b4 = –0.410753	z = –2.236615	P = 0.0253
Religion (4)	b5 = –0.458936	z = –2.956375	P = 0.0031
Ethnic Groups (1)	b6 = –0.372679	z = –2.652628	P = 0.008
Ethnic Groups (2)	b7 = –0.408603	z = –2.811666	P = 0.0049
Ethnic Groups (3)	b8 = –0.008189	z = –0.021336	P = 0.983
Ethnic Groups (4)	b9 = –0.216317	z = –0.780456	P = 0.4351
Ethnic Groups (5)	b10 = –0.236577	z = –0.74567	P = 0.4559
Ethnic Groups (6)	b11 = –0.128619	z = –0.733216	P = 0.4634

logit Ques5 = –1.370984 –0.026447 Age –0.411853 Religion (1) –0.089442 Religion (2) – 0.410753 Religion (3) –0.458936 Religion (4) –0.372679 Ethnic Groups (1) –0.408603 Ethnic Groups (2) –0.008189 Ethnic Groups (3) –0.216317 Ethnic Groups (4) –0.236577 Ethnic Groups (5) –0.128619 Ethnic Groups (6)

Logistic regression – odds ratios

Parameter	Estimate	Odds Ratio	95% CI
Constant	−1.370984		
Age	−0.026447	0.973899	0.753325 to 1.259058
Religion (1)	−0.411853	0.662421	0.537158 to 0.816897
Religion (2)	−0.089442	0.914441	0.700918 to 1.193011
Religion (3)	−0.410753	0.663151	0.46269 to 0.950462
Religion (4)	−0.458936	0.631956	0.466176 to 0.85669
Ethnic Groups (1)	−0.372679	0.688886	0.523068 to 0.90727
Ethnic Groups (2)	−0.408603	0.664578	0.499857 to 0.883581
Ethnic Groups (3)	−0.008189	0.991844	0.467445 to 2.104533
Ethnic Groups (4)	−0.216317	0.80548	0.467875 to 1.386691
Ethnic Groups (5)	−0.236577	0.789325	0.423835 to 1.469992
Ethnic Groups (6)	−0.128619	0.879309	0.623485 to 1.240101

Logistic regression

Warning: result not of full rank, there is more than one solution for the model.

Deviance goodness of fit chi-square =	5.13065	df = 25	P > 0.9999
Deviance (likelihood ratio) chi-square =	1.057635	df = 9	P = 0.9993
Intercept	b0 = −1.462458	z = −8.11211	P < 0.0001
Age	b1 = −0.028214	z = −0.217105	P = 0.8281
Religion (1)	b2 = −0.386177	z = −3.664888	P = 0.0002
Religion (2)	b3 = −0.347967	z = −2.482752	P = 0.013
Religion (3)	b4 = −0.41607	z = −2.293302	P = 0.0218
Religion (4)	b5 = −0.312243	z = −2.123902	P = 0.0337
Ethnic Groups (1)	b6 = −0.200377	z = −1.373546	P = 0.1696
Ethnic Groups (2)	b7 = −0.213166	z = −1.409704	P = 0.1586
Ethnic Groups (3)	b8 = −0.429837	z = −0.943696	P = 0.3453
Ethnic Groups (4)	b9 = −0.110889	z = −0.404716	P = 0.6857
Ethnic Groups (5)	b10 = −0.386754	z = −1.093866	P = 0.274
Ethnic Groups (6)	b11 = −0.121435	z = −0.650201	P = 0.5156

logit Ques6 = −1.462458 −0.028214 Age −0.386177 Religion (1) −0.347967 Religion (2) − 0.41607 Religion (3) −0.312243 Religion (4) −0.200377 Ethnic Groups (1) −0.213166 Ethnic Groups (2) −0.429837 Ethnic Groups (3) −0.110889 Ethnic Groups (4) −0.386754 Ethnic Groups (5) −0.121435 Ethnic Groups (6)

Logistic regression – odds ratios

Parameter	Estimate	Odds Ratio	95% CI
Constant	–1.462458		
Age	–0.028214	0.972181	0.753581 to 1.254193
Religion (1)	–0.386177	0.67965	0.552831 to 0.835561
Religion (2)	–0.347967	0.706122	0.536513 to 0.929349
Religion (3)	–0.41607	0.659634	0.462244 to 0.941316
Religion (4)	–0.312243	0.731803	0.5486 to 0.976187
Ethnic Groups (1)	–0.200377	0.818422	0.614896 to 1.089314
Ethnic Groups (2)	–0.213166	0.808022	0.600773 to 1.086766
Ethnic Groups (3)	–0.429837	0.650615	0.26645 to 1.588663
Ethnic Groups (4)	–0.110889	0.895038	0.523142 to 1.531312
Ethnic Groups (5)	–0.386754	0.679258	0.339686 to 1.358286
Ethnic Groups (6)	–0.121435	0.885649	0.614168 to 1.277133

Logistic regression

Warning: result not of full rank, there is more than one solution for the model.

Deviance goodness of fit chi-square =	23.570029	df = 25	P = 0.5443
Deviance (likelihood ratio) chi-square =	9.169472	df = 9	P = 0.4218
Intercept	b0 = –2.004669	z = –8.176087	P < 0.0001
Age	b1 = –0.072671	z = –0.420905	P = 0.6738
Religion (1)	b2 = –0.373163	z = –2.668591	P = 0.0076
Religion (2)	b3 = –0.759702	z = –3.816393	P = 0.0001
Religion (3)	b4 = –0.764375	z = –2.870872	P = 0.0041
Religion (4)	b5 = –0.107429	z = –0.580935	P = 0.5613
Ethnic Groups (1)	b6 = –0.30597	z = –1.534619	P = 0.1249
Ethnic Groups (2)	b7 = –0.165415	z = –0.802687	P = 0.4222
Ethnic Groups (3)	b8 = –0.593478	z = –0.942249	P = 0.3461
Ethnic Groups (4)	b9 = –0.472799	z = –1.188128	P = 0.2348
Ethnic Groups (5)	b10 = –0.593732	z = –1.13603	P = 0.2559
Ethnic Groups (6)	b11 = 0.126725	z = 0.530241	P = 0.5959

logit Ques7 = –2.004669 –0.072671 Age –0.373163 Religion (1) –0.759702 Religion (2) – 0.764375 Religion (3) –0.107429 Religion (4) –0.30597 Ethnic Groups (1) –0.165415 Ethnic Groups (2) –0.593478 Ethnic Groups (3) –0.472799 Ethnic Groups (4) –0.593732 Ethnic Groups (5) +0.126725 Ethnic Groups (6)

Logistic regression - odds ratios

Parameter	Estimate	Odds Ratio	95% CI
Constant	–2.004669		
Age	–0.072671	0.929907	0.662943 to 1.304375
Religion (1)	–0.373163	0.688553	0.523491 to 0.90566
Religion (2)	–0.759702	0.467806	0.316682 to 0.691048
Religion (3)	–0.764375	0.465625	0.276314 to 0.78464
Religion (4)	–0.107429	0.89814	0.62508 to 1.290484
Ethnic Groups (1)	–0.30597	0.736409	0.498205 to 1.088504
Ethnic Groups (2)	–0.165415	0.847542	0.565911 to 1.269329
Ethnic Groups (3)	–0.593478	0.552402	0.16074 to 1.898399
Ethnic Groups (4)	–0.472799	0.623255	0.285721 to 1.359533
Ethnic Groups (5)	–0.593732	0.552262	0.198278 to 1.53821
Ethnic Groups (6)	0.126725	1.135105	0.710564 to 1.813297

Logistic regression

Warning: result not of full rank, there is more than one solution for the model.

Deviance goodness of fit chi-square =	28.425225	df = 25	P = 0.2887
Deviance (likelihood ratio) chi-square =	62.127401	df = 9	P < 0.0001
Intercept	$b_0 = -3.645717$	z = –0.024668	P = 0.9803
Age	$b_1 = -0.55919$	z = –2.149142	P = 0.0316
Religion (1)	$b_2 = -1.532837$	z = –0.041487	P = 0.9669
Religion (2)	$b_3 = -0.196438$	z = –0.005317	P = 0.9958
Religion (3)	$b_4 = -1.196738$	z = –0.032389	P = 0.9742
Religion (4)	$b_5 = -0.719704$	z = –0.019479	P = 0.9845
Ethnic Groups (1)	$b_6 = 1.348005$	z = 0.007297	P = 0.9942
Ethnic Groups (2)	$b_7 = 1.883376$	z = 0.010195	P = 0.9919
Ethnic Groups (3)	$b_8 = 2.589643$	z = 0.014018	P = 0.9888
Ethnic Groups (4)	$b_9 = -13.257968$	z = –0.012374	P = 0.9901
Ethnic Groups (5)	$b_{10} = 1.165363$	z = 0.006308	P = 0.995
Ethnic Groups (6)	$b_{11} = 2.625864$	z = 0.014214	P = 0.9887

logit Ques8 = –3.645717 –0.55919 Age –1.532837 Religion (1) –0.196438 Religion (2) – 1.196738 Religion (3) –0.719704 Religion (4) +1.348005 Ethnic Groups (1) +1.883376 Ethnic Groups (2) +2.589643 Ethnic Groups (3) –13.257968 Ethnic Groups (4) +1.165363 Ethnic Groups (5) +2.625864 Ethnic Groups (6)

Logistic regression – odds ratios

Parameter	Estimate	Odds Ratio	95% CI
Constant	–3.645717		
Age	–0.55919	0.571672	0.343298 to 0.951969
Religion (1)	–1.532837	0.215922	7.66E–33 to 6.08541909673427E+30
Religion (2)	–0.196438	0.821652	2.92E–32 to 2.31523460055965E+31
Religion (3)	–1.196738	0.302178	1.07E–32 to 8.54123118836728E+30
Religion (4)	–0.719704	0.486896	1.73E–32 to 1.37331928359938E+31
Ethnic Groups (1)	1.348005	3.849737	2.18E–15 to 6.79887583266456E+157
Ethnic Groups (2)	1.883376	6.575667	3.72E–157 to 1.1610728887642E+158
Ethnic Groups (3)	2.589643	13.325008	7.53E–157 to 2.35713703401322E+158
Ethnic Groups (4)	–13.257968	0.000002	* to *
Ethnic Groups (5)	1.165363	3.207088	1.81E–157 to 5.68380078786838E+157
Ethnic Groups (6)	2.625864	13.816509	7.82E–157 to 2.43980382480092E+158

Logistic regression

Warning: rank changed, consider dropping predictors.
Warning: result not of full rank, there is more than one solution for the model.

Deviance goodness of fit chi-square =	24.928145	df = 24	P = 0.4097
Deviance (likelihood ratio) chi-square =	108.616611	df = 10	P < 0.0001
Intercept	b0 = –6.112333	z = –2.68E–14	P > 0.9999
Age	b1 = –0.278099	z = –0.985817	P = 0.3242
Religion (1)	b2 = –2.549066	z = –1.58E–14	P > 0.9999
Religion (2)	b3 = –0.496306	z = –3.07E–15	P > 0.9999
Religion (3)	b4 = –2.21435	z = –1.37E–14	P > 0.9999
Religion (4)	b5 = –0.852611	z = –5.27E–15	P > 0.9999
Ethnic Groups (1)	b6 = 2.861791	z = 4.33E–14	P > 0.9999
Ethnic Groups (2)	b7 = 4.35383	z = 6.58E–14	P > 0.9999
Ethnic Groups (3)	b8 = 4.429242	z = 6.70E–14	P > 0.9999
Ethnic Groups (4)	b9 = –11.826086	z = –1.79E–13	P > 0.9999
Ethnic Groups (5)	b10 = –11.277956	z = –1.71E–13	P > 0.9999
Ethnic Groups (6)	b11 = 5.346848	z = 8.08E–14	P > 0.9999

logit Ques9 = –6.112333 –0.278099 Age –2.549066 Religion (1) –0.496306 Religion (2) – 2.21435 Religion (3) –0.852611 Religion (4) +2.861791 Ethnic Groups (1) +4.35383 Ethnic Groups (2) +4.429242 Ethnic Groups (3) –11.826086 Ethnic Groups (4) –11.277956 Ethnic Groups (5) +5.346848 Ethnic Groups (6)

Logistic regression – odds ratios

Parameter	Estimate	Odds Ratio	95% CI
Constant	–6.112333		
Age	–0.278099	0.757222	0.435612 to 1.316276
Religion (1)	–2.549066	0.078155	* to *
Religion (2)	–0.496306	0.608775	* to *
Religion (3)	–2.21435	0.109225	* to *
Religion (4)	–0.852611	0.4263	* to *
Ethnic Groups (1)	2.861791	17.49282	* to*
Ethnic Groups (2)	4.35383	77.775754	* to *
Ethnic Groups (3)	4.429242	83.867791	* to *
Ethnic Groups (4)	–11.826086	0.000007	* to *
Ethnic Groups (5)	–11.277956	0.000013	* to *
Ethnic Groups (6)	5.346848	209.945472	* to *

Logistic regression

Warning: result not of full rank, there is more than one solution for the model.

Deviance goodness of fit chi-square =	6.134932	df = 25	P > 0.9999
Deviance (likelihood ratio) chi-square =	6.963407	df = 9	P = 0.6409
Intercept	b0 = –1.45819	z = –7.717515	P < 0.0001
Age	b1 = –0.131927	z = –0.94573	P = 0.3443
Religion (1)	b2 = –0.283359	z = –2.48213	P = 0.0131
Religion (2)	b3 = –0.413889	z = –2.575564	P = 0.01
Religion (3)	b4 = –0.379942	z = –1.900462	P = 0.0574
Religion (4)	b5 = –0.381	z = –2.33256	P = 0.0197
Ethnic Groups (1)	b6 = –0.190903	z = –1.301518	P = 0.1931
Ethnic Groups (2)	b7 = –0.338823	z = –2.159054	P = 0.0308
Ethnic Groups (3)	b8 = 0.141851	z = 0.367291	P = 0.7134
Ethnic Groups (4)	b9 = –0.020775	z = –0.073756	P = 0.9412
Ethnic Groups (5)	b10 = –0.469031	z = –1.248139	P = 0.212
Ethnic Groups (6)	b11 = –0.580509	z = –2.670922	P = 0.0076

logit Ques10 = –1.45819 –0.131927 Age –0.283359 Religion (1) –0.413889 Religion (2) – 0.379942 Religion (3) –0.381 Religion (4) –0.190903 Ethnic Groups (1) –0.338823 Ethnic Groups (2) +0.141851 Ethnic Groups (3) –0.020775 Ethnic Groups (4) –0.469031 Ethnic Groups (5) –0.580509 Ethnic Groups (6)

Logistic regression – odds ratios

Parameter	Estimate	Odds Ratio	95% CI
Constant	−1.45819		
Age	−0.131927	0.876405	0.666752 to 1.151981
Religion (1)	−0.283359	0.753249	0.602235 to 0.942132
Religion (2)	−0.413889	0.661074	0.482463 to 0.90581
Religion (3)	−0.379942	0.683901	0.462189 to 1.011967
Religion (4)	−0.381	0.683178	0.496019 to 0.940955
Ethnic Groups (1)	−0.190903	0.826213	0.619784 to 1.101396
Ethnic Groups (2)	−0.338823	0.712609	0.523927 to 0.96924
Ethnic Groups (3)	0.141851	1.152405	0.540585 to 2.456664
Ethnic Groups (4)	−0.020775	0.97944	0.563926 to 1.701114
Ethnic Groups (5)	−0.469031	0.625608	0.299525 to 1.306685
Ethnic Groups (6)	−0.580509	0.559613	0.365497 to 0.856824

Stigma-related Attitudes/ Perceptions – Full Model

Logistic Regression

Warning: result not of full rank, there is more than one solution for the model.

Deviance goodness of fit chi-square =	5.109438	df = 12	P = 0.9542
Deviance (likelihood ratio) chi-square =	3.966116	df = 8	P = 0.8602
Intercept	b0 = –1.857663	z = –14.54692	P < 0.0001
Religious Group (1)	b1 = –0.43871	z = –3.646002	P = 0.0003
Religious Group (2)	b2 = –0.664237	z = –4.008139	P < 0.0001
Religious Group (3)	b3 = –0.363496	z = –1.975057	P = 0.0483
Religious Group (4)	b4 = –0.39122	z = –2.388855	P = 0.0169
Ethnic Group (1)	b5 = –0.125948	z = –0.688661	P = 0.491
Ethnic Group (2)	b6 = –0.221744	z = –1.151888	P = 0.2494
Ethnic Group (3)	b7 = –0.364787	z = –0.574904	P = 0.5654
Ethnic Group (4)	b8 = –0.258792	z = –0.77522	P = 0.4382
Ethnic Group (5)	b9 = –0.740209	z = –1.41955	P = 0.1557
Ethnic Group (6)	b10 = –0.146182	z = –0.644918	P = 0.519

logit Scale = –1.857663 –0.43871 Religious Group (1) –0.664237 Religious Group (2) – 0.363496 Religious Group (3) –0.39122 Religious Group (4) –0.125948 Ethnic Group (1) – 0.221744 Ethnic Group (2) –0.364787 Ethnic Group (3) –0.258792 Ethnic Group (4) – 0.740209 Ethnic Group (5) –0.146182 Ethnic Group (6)

Logistic regression - odds ratios

Parameter	Estimate	Odds Ratio	95% CI
Constant	−1.857663		
Religious Group (1)	−0.43871	0.644868	0.509388 to 0.816381
Religious Group (2)	−0.664237	0.514666	0.371931 to 0.712178
Religious Group (3)	−0.363496	0.695241	0.484705 to 0.997226
Religious Group (4)	−0.39122	0.676232	0.490564 to 0.932171
Ethnic Group (1)	−0.125948	0.88166	0.616065 to 1.261759
Ethnic Group (2)	−0.221744	0.80112	0.549335 to 1.168311
Ethnic Group (3)	−0.364787	0.694344	0.200203 to 2.408122
Ethnic Group (4)	−0.258792	0.771983	0.401283 to 1.485132
Ethnic Group (5)	−0.740209	0.477014	0.171665 to 1.325504
Ethnic Group (6)	−0.146182	0.864	0.554082 to 1.347268

The Thirteen HIV and AIDS Stigma-related Attitude/Perception Items

Logistic regression

Warning: result not of full rank, there is more than one solution for the model.

Deviance goodness of fit chi-square =	9.391207	df = 12	P = 0.6692
Deviance (likelihood ratio) chi-square =	11.694701	df = 8	P = 0.1654
Intercept	b0 = −1.680339	z = −15.535248	P < 0.0001
Religion (1)	b1 = −0.527242	z = −4.399716	P < 0.0001
Religion (2)	b2 = −0.251429	z = −1.75866	P = 0.0786
Religion (3)	b3 = −0.596477	z = −3.106655	P = 0.0019
Religion (4)	b4 = −0.305191	z = −1.903338	P = 0.057
Ethnic Groups (1)	b5 = −0.553663	z = −3.263778	P = 0.0011
Ethnic Groups (2)	b6 = −0.30388	z = −1.79397	P = 0.0728
Ethnic Groups (3)	b7 = −0.054087	z = −0.10233	P = 0.9185
Ethnic Groups (4)	b8 = −0.541189	z = −1.596284	P = 0.1104
Ethnic Groups (5)	b9 = −0.113759	z = −0.295589	P = 0.7675
Ethnic Groups (6)	b10 = −0.113761	z = −0.574731	P = 0.5655

logit Ques1 = −1.680339 −0.527242 Religion (1) −0.251429 Religion (2) −0.596477 Religion (3) −0.305191 Religion (4) −0.553663 Ethnic Groups (1) −0.30388 Ethnic Groups (2) −0.054087 Ethnic Groups (3) −0.541189 Ethnic Groups (4) −0.113759 Ethnic Groups (5) −0.113761 Ethnic Groups (6)

Logistic regression – odds ratios

Parameter	Estimate	Odds Ratio	95% CI
Constant	−1.680339		
Religion (1)	−0.527242	0.590231	0.466678 to 0.746493
Religion (2)	−0.251429	0.777688	0.587641 to 1.029198
Religion (3)	−0.596477	0.550749	0.378027 to 0.802387
Religion (4)	−0.305191	0.736983	0.538234 to 1.009121
Ethnic Groups (1)	−0.553663	0.57484	0.41224 to 0.801575
Ethnic Groups (2)	−0.30388	0.737949	0.52947 to 1.028517
Ethnic Groups (3)	−0.054087	0.94735	0.336204 to 2.669424
Ethnic Groups (4)	−0.541189	0.582056	0.299489 to 1.131222
Ethnic Groups (5)	−0.113759	0.892473	0.419765 to 1.897512
Ethnic Groups (6)	−0.113761	0.892472	0.605494 to 1.315463

Logistic regression

Warning: result not of full rank, there is more than one solution for the model.

Deviance goodness of fit chi-square =	6.284508	df = 12	P = 0.9011
Deviance (likelihood ratio) chi-square =	8.499219	df = 8	P = 0.3863
Intercept	$b_0 = -1.741583$	$z = -16.423408$	P < 0.0001
Religion (1)	$b_1 = -0.605125$	$z = -4.564125$	P < 0.0001
Religion (2)	$b_2 = -0.211235$	$z = -1.324687$	P = 0.1853
Religion (3)	$b_3 = -0.540932$	$z = -2.619178$	P = 0.0088
Religion (4)	$b_4 = -0.384291$	$z = -2.181586$	P = 0.0291
Ethnic Groups (1)	$b_5 = -0.535244$	$z = -3.097132$	P = 0.002
Ethnic Groups (2)	$b_6 = -0.473297$	$z = -2.683717$	P = 0.0073
Ethnic Groups (3)	$b_7 = 0.398621$	$z = 0.847811$	P = 0.3965
Ethnic Groups (4)	$b_8 = -0.561879$	$z = -1.573902$	P = 0.1155
Ethnic Groups (5)	$b_9 = -0.005939$	$z = -0.015455$	P = 0.9877
Ethnic Groups (6)	$b_{10} = -0.563845$	$z = -2.490975$	P = 0.0127

logit Ques2 = −1.741583 −0.605125 Religion (1) −0.211235 Religion (2) −0.540932 Religion (3) −0.384291 Religion (4) −0.535244 Ethnic Groups (1) −0.473297 Ethnic Groups (2) +0.398621 Ethnic Groups (3) −0.561879 Ethnic Groups (4) −0.005939 Ethnic Groups (5) −0.563845 Ethnic Groups (6)

Logistic regression – odds ratios

Parameter	Estimate	Odds Ratio	95% CI		
Constant	–1.741583				
Religion (1)	–0.605125	0.546006	0.421059	to	0.708031
Religion (2)	–0.211235	0.809584	0.592282	to	1.10661
Religion (3)	–0.540932	0.582205	0.3884	to	0.872715
Religion (4)	–0.384291	0.680933	0.482129	to	0.961713
Ethnic Groups (1)	–0.535244	0.585526	0.417294	to	0.821581
Ethnic Groups (2)	–0.473297	0.622945	0.440893	to	0.88017
Ethnic Groups (3)	0.398621	1.48977	0.592794	to	3.74399
Ethnic Groups (4)	–0.561879	0.570137	0.283206	to	1.147772
Ethnic Groups (5)	–0.005939	0.994079	0.468085	to	2.111141
Ethnic Groups (6)	–0.563845	0.569017	0.365133	to	0.886745

Logistic regression

Warning: result not of full rank, there is more than one solution for the model.

Deviance goodness of fit chi-square =	23.435438	df = 12	P = 0.0242*
Deviance (likelihood ratio) chi-square =	21.851406	df = 8	P = 0.0052
Intercept	b0 = –4.518386	z = –0.030817	P = 0.9754
Religion (1)	b1 = –2.153724	z = –0.058753	P = 0.9531
Religion (2)	b2 = –0.454606	z = –0.012402	P = 0.9901
Religion (3)	b3 = –1.161459	z = –0.031683	P = 0.9747
Religion (4)	b4 = –0.748596	z = –0.020422	P = 0.9837
Ethnic Groups (1)	b5 = 1.096128	z = 0.005981	P = 0.9952
Ethnic Groups (2)	b6 = 0.859744	z = 0.004691	P = 0.9963
Ethnic Groups (3)	b7 = 3.324595	z = 0.01814	P = 0.9855
Ethnic Groups (4)	b8 = –13.373329	z = –0.012581	P = 0.99
Ethnic Groups (5)	b9 = 2.014475	z = 0.010991	P = 0.9912
Ethnic Groups (6)	b10 = 1.560001	z = 0.008512	P = 0.9932

logit Ques3 = –4.518386 –2.153724 Religion (1) –0.454606 Religion (2) –1.161459 Religion (3) –0.748596 Religion (4) +1.096128 Ethnic Groups (1) +0.859744 Ethnic Groups (2) +3.324595 Ethnic Groups (3) –13.373329 Ethnic Groups (4) +2.014475 Ethnic Groups (5) +1.560001 Ethnic Groups (6)

Logistic regression – odds ratios

Parameter	Estimate	Odds Ratio	95% CI
Constant	–4.518386		
Religion (1)	–2.153724	0.116051	7.28E–33 to 1.85015196592506E+30
Religion (2)	–0.454606	0.634698	3.98E–32 to 1.01138312893142E+31
Religion (3)	–1.161459	0.313029	1.96E–32 to 5.00327041625645E+30
Religion (4)	–0.748596	0.47303	2.97E–32 to 7.5411062722495E+30
Ethnic Groups (1)	1.096128	2.992557	2.96E–156 to 3.02526794140502E+156
Ethnic Groups (2)	0.859744	2.362556	2.34E–156 to 2.38801075797809E+156
Ethnic Groups (3)	3.324595	27.787748	2.74E–155 to 2.81334688935216E+157
Ethnic Groups (4)	–13.373329	0.000002	* to *
Ethnic Groups (5)	2.014475	7.496789	7.39E–156 to 7.60372896483433E+156
Ethnic Groups (6)	1.560001	4.758824	4.71E–156 to 4.81120329407476E+156

Logistic regression

Warning: result not of full rank, there is more than one solution for the model.

Deviance goodness of fit chi-square =	10.723329	df = 12	P = 0.5528
Deviance (likelihood ratio) chi-square =	10.383497	df = 8	P = 0.2391
Intercept	b0 = –6.066808	z = –0.012214	P = 0.9903
Religion (1)	b1 = 2.007078	z = 0.003464	P = 0.9972
Religion (2)	b2 = 3.414565	z = 0.005892	P = 0.9953
Religion (3)	b3 = –13.93547	z = –0.006235	P = 0.995
Religion (4)	b4 = 2.44702	z = 0.004223	P = 0.9966
Ethnic Groups (1)	b5 = –1.191594	z = –0.014394	P = 0.9885
Ethnic Groups (2)	b6 = –1.96784	z = –0.02377	P = 0.981
Ethnic Groups (3)	b7 = 0.634348	z = 0.007662	P = 0.9939
Ethnic Groups (4)	b8 = –0.831642	z = –0.010045	P = 0.992
Ethnic Groups (5)	b9 = –0.238094	z = –0.002876	P = 0.9977
Ethnic Groups (6)	b10 = –2.471987	z = –0.029859	P = 0.9762

logit Ques4 = –6.066808 +2.007078 Religion (1) +3.414565 Religion (2) –13.93547 Religion (3) +2.44702 Religion (4) –1.191594 Ethnic Groups (1) –1.96784 Ethnic Groups (2) +0.634348 Ethnic Groups (3) –0.831642 Ethnic Groups (4) –0.238094 Ethnic Groups (5) –2.471987 Ethnic Groups (6)

Logistic regression – odds ratios

Parameter	Estimate	Odds Ratio	95% CI
Constant	−6.066808		
Religion (1)	2.007078	7.441538	* to *
Religion (2)	3.414565	30.403706	* to *
Religion (3)	−13.93547	8.87E−07	* to *
Religion (4)	2.44702	11.553864	* to *
Ethnic Groups (1)	−1.191594	0.303737	1.04E−71 to 8.89397438874087E+69
Ethnic Groups (2)	−1.96784	0.139758	4.77E−72 to 4.09793605577789E+69
Ethnic Groups (3)	0.634348	1.885792	6.39E−71 to 5.56344855677389E+70
Ethnic Groups (4)	−0.831642	0.435334	1.48E−71 to 1.28470217361982E+70
Ethnic Groups (5)	−0.238094	0.788129	2.67E−71 to 2.32390892219996E+70
Ethnic Groups (6)	−2.471987	0.084417	2.86E−72 to 2.49028297294259E+69

Logistic regression

Warning: result not of full rank, there is more than one solution for the model.

Deviance goodness of fit chi-square =	8.889519	df = 12	P = 0.7123
Deviance (likelihood ratio) chi-square =	7.218675	df = 8	P = 0.5132
Intercept	$b0 = -1.542249$	$z = -16.31313$	P < 0.0001
Religion (1)	$b1 = -0.460211$	$z = -3.941433$	P < 0.0001
Religion (2)	$b2 = -0.184241$	$z = -1.260348$	P = 0.2075
Religion (3)	$b3 = -0.495769$	$z = -2.638821$	P = 0.0083
Religion (4)	$b4 = -0.402028$	$z = -2.476416$	P = 0.0133
Ethnic Groups (1)	$b5 = -0.487366$	$z = -3.234915$	P = 0.0012
Ethnic Groups (2)	$b6 = -0.553748$	$z = -3.487609$	P = 0.0005
Ethnic Groups (3)	$b7 = 0.378806$	$z = 0.885938$	P = 0.3757
Ethnic Groups (4)	$b8 = -0.541483$	$z = -1.707933$	P = 0.0876
Ethnic Groups (5)	$b9 = 0.133895$	$z = 0.413368$	P = 0.6793
Ethnic Groups (6)	$b10 = -0.472353$	$z = -2.419016$	P = 0.0156

logit Ques5 = −1.542249 −0.460211 Religion (1) −0.184241 Religion (2) −0.495769 Religion (3) −0.402028 Religion (4) −0.487366 Ethnic Groups (1) −0.553748 Ethnic Groups (2) +0.378806 Ethnic Groups (3) −0.541483 Ethnic Groups (4) +0.133895 Ethnic Groups (5) −0.472353 Ethnic Groups (6)

Logistic regression – odds ratios

Parameter	Estimate	Odds Ratio	95% CI
Constant	–1.542249		
Religion (1)	–0.460211	0.63115	0.502047 to 0.793453
Religion (2)	–0.184241	0.831735	0.624532 to 1.107684
Religion (3)	–0.495769	0.609102	0.421474 to 0.880258
Religion (4)	–0.402028	0.668962	0.486648 to 0.919576
Ethnic Groups (1)	–0.487366	0.614242	0.457193 to 0.82524
Ethnic Groups (2)	–0.553748	0.574792	0.421076 to 0.784622
Ethnic Groups (3)	0.378806	1.46054	0.631771 to 3.376502
Ethnic Groups (4)	–0.541483	0.581885	0.312588 to 1.083183
Ethnic Groups (5)	0.133895	1.143273	0.605948 to 2.157072
Ethnic Groups (6)	–0.472353	0.623533	0.425254 to 0.914263

Logistic regression

Warning: result not of full rank, there is more than one solution for the model.

Deviance goodness of fit chi-square =	5.485809	df = 12	P = 0.9398
Deviance (likelihood ratio) chi-square =	3.639409	df = 8	P = 0.8881
Intercept	$b_0 = -1.324591$	$z = -15.490073$	P < 0.0001
Religion (1)	$b_1 = -0.351219$	$z = -3.566257$	P = 0.0004
Religion (2)	$b_2 = -0.299928$	$z = -2.374058$	P = 0.0176
Religion (3)	$b_3 = -0.385086$	$z = -2.478918$	P = 0.0132
Religion (4)	$b_4 = -0.288359$	$z = -2.123698$	P = 0.0337
Ethnic Groups (1)	$b_5 = -0.457284$	$z = -3.432056$	P = 0.0006
Ethnic Groups (2)	$b_6 = -0.356292$	$z = -2.584256$	P = 0.0098
Ethnic Groups (3)	$b_7 = 0.273725$	$z = 0.688801$	P = 0.4909
Ethnic Groups (4)	$b_8 = -0.30469$	$z = -1.183814$	P = 0.2365
Ethnic Groups (5)	$b_9 = -0.170206$	$z = -0.532295$	P = 0.5945
Ethnic Groups (6)	$b_{10} = -0.309844$	$z = -1.834373$	P = 0.0666

logit Ques6 = –1.324591 –0.351219 Religion (1) –0.299928 Religion (2) –0.385086 Religion (3) –0.288359 Religion (4) –0.457284 Ethnic Groups (1) –0.356292 Ethnic Groups (2) +0.273725 Ethnic Groups (3) –0.30469 Ethnic Groups (4) –0.170206 Ethnic Groups (5) –0.309844 Ethnic Groups (6)

Logistic regression – odds ratios

Parameter	Estimate	Odds Ratio	95% CI
Constant	−1.324591		
Religion (1)	−0.351219	0.70383	0.580281 to 0.853684
Religion (2)	−0.299928	0.740872	0.578371 to 0.94903
Religion (3)	−0.385086	0.680392	0.501799 to 0.922547
Religion (4)	−0.288359	0.749493	0.574368 to 0.978013
Ethnic Groups (1)	−0.457284	0.633	0.487518 to 0.821897
Ethnic Groups (2)	−0.356292	0.700268	0.534452 to 0.917529
Ethnic Groups (3)	0.273725	1.314854	0.603414 to 2.865099
Ethnic Groups (4)	−0.30469	0.737352	0.445239 to 1.221116
Ethnic Groups (5)	−0.170206	0.843491	0.450714 to 1.578555
Ethnic Groups (6)	−0.309844	0.733561	0.526817 to 1.02144

Logistic regression

Warning: result not of full rank, there is more than one solution for the model.

Deviance goodness of fit chi-square =	2.053689	df = 12	P = 0.9993
Deviance (likelihood ratio) chi-square =	2.985531	df = 8	P = 0.9353
Intercept	$b0 = -1.296328$	$z = -15.238468$	P < 0.0001
Religion (1)	$b1 = -0.39094$	$z = -4.008148$	P < 0.0001
Religion (2)	$b2 = -0.223215$	$z = -1.800217$	P = 0.0718
Religion (3)	$b3 = -0.37661$	$z = -2.45622$	P = 0.014
Religion (4)	$b4 = -0.305563$	$z = -2.28787$	P = 0.0221
Ethnic Groups (1)	$b5 = -0.346823$	$z = -2.636044$	P = 0.0084
Ethnic Groups (2)	$b6 = -0.36755$	$z = -2.672777$	P = 0.0075
Ethnic Groups (3)	$b7 = 0.273484$	$z = 0.688124$	P = 0.4914
Ethnic Groups (4)	$b8 = -0.3111$	$z = -1.209169$	P = 0.2266
Ethnic Groups (5)	$b9 = -0.176607$	$z = -0.552456$	P = 0.5806
Ethnic Groups (6)	$b10 = -0.367731$	$z = -2.161723$	P = 0.0306

logit Ques7 = −1.296328 −0.39094 Religion (1) −0.223215 Religion (2) −0.37661 Religion (3) −0.305563 Religion (4) −0.346823 Ethnic Groups (1) −0.36755 Ethnic Groups (2) +0.273484 Ethnic Groups (3) −0.3111 Ethnic Groups (4) −0.176607 Ethnic Groups (5) −0.367731 Ethnic Groups (6)

Logistic regression – odds ratios

Parameter	Estimate	Odds Ratio	95% CI		
Constant	−1.296328				
Religion (1)	−0.39094	0.676421	0.55872	to	0.818917
Religion (2)	−0.223215	0.799943	0.627358	to	1.020005
Religion (3)	−0.37661	0.686183	0.508073	to	0.926732
Religion (4)	−0.305563	0.736709	0.567037	to	0.957151
Ethnic Groups (1)	−0.346823	0.70693	0.546241	to	0.91489
Ethnic Groups (2)	−0.36755	0.692429	0.528836	to	0.906628
Ethnic Groups (3)	0.273484	1.314537	0.60322	to	2.864638
Ethnic Groups (4)	−0.3111	0.73264	0.442476	to	1.213087
Ethnic Groups (5)	−0.176607	0.838109	0.44791	to	1.56823
Ethnic Groups (6)	−0.367731	0.692303	0.496019	to	0.966261

Logistic regression

Warning: result not of full rank, there is more than one solution for the model.

Deviance goodness of fit chi-square =	9.054456	df = 12	P = 0.6983
Deviance (likelihood ratio) chi-square =	6.806756	df = 8	P = 0.5576
Intercept	$b0 = -6.924007$	$z = -0.010536$	P = 0.9916
Religion (1)	$b1 = -2.166853$	$z = -0.013189$	P = 0.9895
Religion (2)	$b2 = -1.291777$	$z = -0.007863$	P = 0.9937
Religion (3)	$b3 = -2.063503$	$z = -0.01256$	P = 0.99
Religion (4)	$b4 = -1.401874$	$z = -0.008533$	P = 0.9932
Ethnic Groups (1)	$b5 = 4.297609$	$z = 0.005232$	P = 0.9958
Ethnic Groups (2)	$b6 = 4.000622$	$z = 0.00487$	P = 0.9961
Ethnic Groups (3)	$b7 = -11.283704$	$z = -0.003139$	P = 0.9975
Ethnic Groups (4)	$b8 = -12.591781$	$z = -0.003895$	P = 0.9969
Ethnic Groups (5)	$b9 = 4.785491$	$z = 0.005826$	P = 0.9954
Ethnic Groups (6)	$b10 = 3.867756$	$z = 0.004709$	P = 0.9962

logit Ques8 = −6.924007 −2.166853 Religion (1) −1.291777 Religion (2) −2.063503 Religion (3) −1.401874 Religion (4) +4.297609 Ethnic Groups (1) +4.000622 Ethnic Groups (2) −11.283704 Ethnic Groups (3) −12.591781 Ethnic Groups (4) +4.785491 Ethnic Groups (5) +3.867756 Ethnic Groups (6)

Logistic regression – odds ratios

Parameter	Estimate	Odds Ratio	95% CI
Constant	–6.924007		
Religion (1)	–2.166853	0.114537	1.65E–141 to 7.96098554632178E+138
Religion (2)	–1.291777	0.274782	3.95E–141 to 1.91018394569783E+139
Religion (3)	–2.063503	0.127008	1.82E–141 to 8.83965785673254E+138
Religion (4)	–1.401874	0.246135	3.54E–141 to 1.71117359994497E+139
Ethnic Groups (1)	4.297609	73.523813	* to *
Ethnic Groups (2)	4.000622	54.632105	* to *
Ethnic Groups (3)	–11.283704	0.000013	* to *
Ethnic Groups (4)	–12.591781	0.000003	* to *
Ethnic Groups (5)	4.785491	119.760122	* to *
Ethnic Groups (6)	3.867756	47.834942	* to *

Logistic regression

Warning: result not of full rank, there is more than one solution for the model.

Deviance goodness of fit chi-square =	7.348326	df = 12	P = 0.8338
Deviance (likelihood ratio) chi-square =	10.241728	df = 8	P = 0.2485
Intercept	b0 = –1.9987	z = –16.249553	P < 0.0001
Religion (1)	b1 = –0.553599	z = –3.516518	P = 0.0004
Religion (2)	b2 = –0.157799	z = –0.842789	P = 0.3993
Religion (3)	b3 = –0.929724	z = –3.30274	P = 0.001
Religion (4)	b4 = –0.357579	z = –1.72549	P = 0.0844
Ethnic Groups (1)	b5 = –0.696859	z = –3.522595	P = 0.0004
Ethnic Groups (2)	b6 = –0.565866	z = –2.793872	P = 0.0052
Ethnic Groups (3)	b7 = 0.32417	z = 0.608637	P = 0.5428
Ethnic Groups (4)	b8 = –0.45326	z = –1.168863	P = 0.2425
Ethnic Groups (5)	b9 = 0.052078	z = 0.124082	P = 0.9013
Ethnic Groups (6)	b10 = –0.658963	z = –2.531848	P = 0.0113

logit Ques9 = –1.9987 –0.553599 Religion (1) –0.157799 Religion (2) –0.929724 Religion (3) –0.357579 Religion (4) –0.696859 Ethnic Groups (1) –0.565866 Ethnic Groups (2) +0.32417 Ethnic Groups (3) –0.45326 Ethnic Groups (4) +0.052078 Ethnic Groups (5) –0.658963 Ethnic Groups (6)

Logistic regression – odds ratios

Parameter	Estimate	Odds Ratio	95% CI		
Constant	−1.9987				
Religion (1)	−0.553599	0.574877	0.422252	to	0.782669
Religion (2)	−0.157799	0.854021	0.591691	to	1.232659
Religion (3)	−0.929724	0.394663	0.227307	to	0.685236
Religion (4)	−0.357579	0.699368	0.465917	to	1.049791
Ethnic Groups (1)	−0.696859	0.498148	0.33804	to	0.734087
Ethnic Groups (2)	−0.565866	0.567868	0.381809	to	0.844595
Ethnic Groups (3)	0.32417	1.382883	0.486879	to	3.9278
Ethnic Groups (4)	−0.45326	0.635553	0.297218	to	1.359031
Ethnic Groups (5)	0.052078	1.053458	0.462769	to	2.398115
Ethnic Groups (6)	−0.658963	0.517387	0.310652	to	0.861703

Logistic regression

Warning: result not of full rank, there is more than one solution for the model.

Deviance goodness of fit chi-square =	13.749782	df = 12	P = 0.317
Deviance (likelihood ratio) chi-square =	10.461995	df = 8	P = 0.2341
Intercept	b0 = −2.219321	z = −16.374859	P < 0.0001
Religion (1)	b1 = −0.858178	z = −4.319272	P < 0.0001
Religion (2)	b2 = −0.441649	z = −1.764359	P = 0.0777
Religion (3)	b3 = −0.371997	z = −1.338713	P = 0.1807
Religion (4)	b4 = −0.547497	z = −2.098253	P = 0.0359
Ethnic Groups (1)	b5 = −0.732913	z = −3.006788	P = 0.0026
Ethnic Groups (2)	b6 = −0.900591	z = −3.532453	P = 0.0004
Ethnic Groups (3)	b7 = 1.0518	z = 2.172607	P = 0.0298
Ethnic Groups (4)	b8 = −0.828681	z = −1.572503	P = 0.1158
Ethnic Groups (5)	b9 = −0.089204	z = −0.16914	P = 0.8657
Ethnic Groups (6)	b10 = −0.719731	z = −2.251738	P = 0.0243

logit Ques10 = −2.219321 −0.858178 Religion (1) −0.441649 Religion (2) −0.371997 Religion (3) −0.547497 Religion (4) −0.732913 Ethnic Groups (1) −0.900591 Ethnic Groups (2) +1.0518 Ethnic Groups (3) −0.828681 Ethnic Groups (4) −0.089204 Ethnic Groups (5) −0.719731 Ethnic Groups (6)

Logistic regression – odds ratios

Parameter	Estimate	Odds Ratio	95% CI	
Constant	−2.219321			
Religion (1)	−0.858178	0.423934	0.287195 to	0.625777
Religion (2)	−0.441649	0.642975	0.393663 to	1.050182
Religion (3)	−0.371997	0.689356	0.399866 to	1.188428
Religion (4)	−0.547497	0.578396	0.346834 to	0.96456
Ethnic Groups (1)	−0.732913	0.480507	0.298001 to	0.774788
Ethnic Groups (2)	−0.900591	0.406329	0.246528 to	0.669715
Ethnic Groups (3)	1.0518	2.862798	1.10843 to	7.393895
Ethnic Groups (4)	−0.828681	0.436625	0.155432 to	1.226525
Ethnic Groups (5)	−0.089204	0.914659	0.32534 to	2.571468
Ethnic Groups (6)	−0.719731	0.486883	0.260227 to	0.910956

Logistic regression

Warning: result not of full rank, there is more than one solution for the model.

Deviance goodness of fit chi-square =	17.57212	df = 12	P = 0.1293
Deviance (likelihood ratio) chi-square =	23.150529	df = 8	P = 0.0032
Intercept	$b0 = -2.39598$	$z = -15.392891$	P < 0.0001
Religion (1)	$b1 = -1.099555$	$z = -4.436968$	P < 0.0001
Religion (2)	$b2 = 0.04135$	$z = 0.155257$	P = 0.8766
Religion (3)	$b3 = -0.638857$	$z = -1.816635$	P = 0.0693
Religion (4)	$b4 = -0.698917$	$z = -2.181814$	P = 0.0291
Ethnic Groups (1)	$b5 = -1.010838$	$z = -3.244606$	P = 0.0012
Ethnic Groups (2)	$b6 = -1.018087$	$z = -3.436799$	P = 0.0006
Ethnic Groups (3)	$b7 = 1.442018$	$z = 2.898226$	P = 0.0038
Ethnic Groups (4)	$b8 = -0.866852$	$z = -1.349523$	P = 0.1772
Ethnic Groups (5)	$b9 = -0.204882$	$z = -0.320622$	P = 0.7485
Ethnic Groups (6)	$b10 = -0.737337$	$z = -2.078548$	P = 0.0377

logit Ques11 = −2.39598 −1.099555 Religion (1) +0.04135 Religion (2) −0.638857 Religion (3) −0.698917 Religion (4) −1.010838 Ethnic Groups (1) −1.018087 Ethnic Groups (2) +1.442018 Ethnic Groups (3) −0.866852 Ethnic Groups (4) −0.204882 Ethnic Groups (5) −0.737337 Ethnic Groups (6)

Logistic regression – odds ratios

Parameter	Estimate	Odds Ratio	95% CI
Constant	−2.39598		
Religion (1)	−1.099555	0.333019	0.204893 to 0.541267
Religion (2)	0.04135	1.042217	0.618382 to 1.756543
Religion (3)	−0.638857	0.527895	0.264975 to 1.051696
Religion (4)	−0.698917	0.497123	0.265334 to 0.931399
Ethnic Groups (1)	−1.010838	0.363914	0.197611 to 0.670171
Ethnic Groups (2)	−1.018087	0.361285	0.202161 to 0.645659
Ethnic Groups (3)	1.442018	4.229221	1.594937 to 11.214435
Ethnic Groups (4)	−0.866852	0.420272	0.119336 to 1.480102
Ethnic Groups (5)	−0.204882	0.814743	0.232857 to 2.850707
Ethnic Groups (6)	−0.737337	0.478386	0.238685 to 0.958807

Logistic regression

Warning: result not of full rank, there is more than one solution for the model.

Deviance goodness of fit chi-square =	8.75289	df = 12	P = 0.7239
Deviance (likelihood ratio) chi-square =	27.397474	df = 8	P = 0.0006
Intercept	$b0 = -2.042428$	$z = -15.519539$	P < 0.0001
Religion (1)	$b1 = -0.775635$	$z = -4.48518$	P < 0.0001
Religion (2)	$b2 = 0.054221$	$z = 0.283581$	P = 0.7767
Religion (3)	$b3 = -0.622137$	$z = -2.368681$	P = 0.0179
Religion (4)	$b4 = -0.698878$	$z = -2.857601$	P = 0.0043
Ethnic Groups (1)	$b5 = -0.700267$	$z = -3.114387$	P = 0.0018
Ethnic Groups (2)	$b6 = -0.626475$	$z = -2.821357$	P = 0.0048
Ethnic Groups (3)	$b7 = 1.169361$	$z = 2.634108$	P = 0.0084
Ethnic Groups (4)	$b8 = -1.328267$	$z = -2.122352$	P = 0.0338
Ethnic Groups (5)	$b9 = 0.192962$	$z = 0.452647$	P = 0.6508
Ethnic Groups (6)	$b10 = -0.749743$	$z = -2.636026$	P = 0.0084

logit Ques12 = −2.042428 −0.775635 Religion (1) +0.054221 Religion (2) −0.622137 Religion (3) −0.698878 Religion (4) −0.700267 Ethnic Groups (1) −0.626475 Ethnic Groups (2) +1.169361 Ethnic Groups (3) −1.328267 Ethnic Groups (4) +0.192962 Ethnic Groups (5) −0.749743 Ethnic Groups (6)

Logistic regression - odds ratios

Parameter	Estimate	Odds Ratio	95% CI
Constant	–2.042428		
Religion (1)	–0.775635	0.460412	0.328054 to 0.64617
Religion (2)	0.054221	1.055718	0.725766 to 1.535676
Religion (3)	–0.622137	0.536796	0.320804 to 0.898211
Religion (4)	–0.698878	0.497143	0.307825 to 0.802893
Ethnic Groups (1)	–0.700267	0.496453	0.319511 to 0.771383
Ethnic Groups (2)	–0.626475	0.534473	0.345875 to 0.82591
Ethnic Groups (3)	1.169361	3.219935	1.348878 to 7.686375
Ethnic Groups (4)	–1.328267	0.264936	0.0777 to 0.903364
Ethnic Groups (5)	0.192962	1.212837	0.525941 to 2.796839
Ethnic Groups (6)	–0.749743	0.472488	0.270577 to 0.82507

Logistic regression

Warning: result not of full rank, there is more than one solution for the model.

Deviance goodness of fit chi-square =	13.105579	df = 12	P = 0.3614
Deviance (likelihood ratio) chi-square =	13.536575	df = 8	P = 0.0947
Intercept	b0 = –1.831054	z = –16.742476	P < 0.0001
Religion (1)	b1 = –0.347408	z = –2.528846	P = 0.0114
Religion (2)	b2 = –0.17024	z = –1.010271	P = 0.3124
Religion (3)	b3 = –0.927626	z = –3.630286	P = 0.0003
Religion (4)	b4 = –0.38578	z = –2.015027	P = 0.0439
Ethnic Groups (1)	b5 = –0.682479	z = –4.002722	P < 0.0001
Ethnic Groups (2)	b6 = –0.500445	z = –2.83093	P = 0.0046
Ethnic Groups (3)	b7 = 0.629268	z = 1.458333	P = 0.1447
Ethnic Groups (4)	b8 = –0.686466	z = –1.810743	P = 0.0702
Ethnic Groups (5)	b9 = 0.093528	z = 0.258884	P = 0.7957
Ethnic Groups (6)	b10 = –0.684459	z = –2.960596	P = 0.0031

logit Ques13 = –1.831054 –0.347408 Religion (1) –0.17024 Religion (2) –0.927626 Religion (3) –0.38578 Religion (4) –0.682479 Ethnic Groups (1) –0.500445 Ethnic Groups (2) +0.629268 Ethnic Groups (3) –0.686466 Ethnic Groups (4) +0.093528 Ethnic Groups (5) –0.684459 Ethnic Groups (6)

Logistic regression – odds ratios

Parameter	Estimate	Odds Ratio	95% CI		
Constant	−1.831054				
Religion (1)	−0.347408	0.706517	0.539742	to	0.924824
Religion (2)	−0.17024	0.843463	0.606221	to	1.173548
Religion (3)	−0.927626	0.395491	0.239681	to	0.652589
Religion (4)	−0.38578	0.67992	0.46719	to	0.989514
Ethnic Groups (1)	−0.682479	0.505362	0.361801	to	0.705888
Ethnic Groups (2)	−0.500445	0.606261	0.428732	to	0.8573
Ethnic Groups (3)	0.629268	1.876237	0.805371	to	4.370986
Ethnic Groups (4)	−0.686466	0.503352	0.239428	to	1.058201
Ethnic Groups (5)	0.093528	1.098041	0.540883	to	2.229119
Ethnic Groups (6)	−0.684459	0.504363	0.320593	to	0.793473

Relationship between HIV and AIDS Knowledge and Stigma-related Perceptions

Logistic regression

Deviance goodness of fit chi-square =	91.475211	df = 48	P = 0.0002*
Deviance (likelihood ratio) chi-square =	21.108756	df = 10	P = 0.0203
Intercept	b0 = 0.192683	z = 0.208582	P = 0.8348
Ques1	b1 = 0.42525	z = 0.690383	P = 0.49
Ques2	b2 = -0.010518	z = -0.021764	P = 0.9826
Ques3	b3 = -0.200011	z = -0.291389	P = 0.7708
Ques4	b4 = 0.78982	z = 1.135988	P = 0.256
Ques5	b5 = -0.818209	z = -2.557715	P = 0.0105
Ques6	b6 = -0.525956	z = -1.450359	P = 0.147
Ques7	b7 = -0.080754	z = -0.354572	P = 0.7229
Ques8	b8 = 0.555596	z = 1.321227	P = 0.1864
Ques9	b9 = 0.582731	z = 0.924542	P = 0.3552
Ques10	b10 = 0.045366	z = 0.165197	P = 0.8688

logit Y = 0.192683 +0.42525 Ques1 –0.010518 Ques2 –0.200011 Ques3 +0.78982 Ques4
–0.818209 Ques5 –0.525956 Ques6 –0.080754 Ques7 +0.555596 Ques8 +0.582731 Ques9
+0.045366 Ques10

Logistic regression – odds ratios

Parameter	Estimate	Odds Ratio	95% CI
Constant	0.192683		
Ques1	0.42525	1.529973	0.457483 to 5.116726
Ques2	–0.010518	0.989537	0.383775 to 2.551455
Ques3	–0.200011	0.818722	0.213239 to 3.143442
Ques4	0.78982	2.202999	0.563895 to 8.606572
Ques5	–0.818209	0.441221	0.235699 to 0.825951
Ques6	–0.525956	0.59099	0.290337 to 1.202981
Ques7	–0.080754	0.922421	0.590294 to 1.441418
Ques8	0.555596	1.742979	0.76445 to 3.974066
Ques9	0.582731	1.790923	0.520681 to 6.160024
Ques10	0.045366	1.046411	0.610868 to 1.79249

Logistic regression

Deviance goodness of fit chi-square =	60.093002	df = 48	P = 0.1131
Deviance (likelihood ratio) chi-square =	13.808963	df = 10	P = 0.1819
Intercept	b0 = −0.278368	z = −0.306925	P = 0.7589
Ques1	b1 = −0.097036	z = −0.167111	P = 0.8673
Ques2	b2 = −0.515647	z = −1.099965	P = 0.2713
Ques3	b3 = 0.222503	z = 0.347589	P = 0.7281
Ques4	b4 = 0.670263	z = 0.940988	P = 0.3467
Ques5	b5 = 0.299508	z = 1.018069	P = 0.3086
Ques6	b6 = −0.373571	z = −1.099782	P = 0.2714
Ques7	b7 = −0.105121	z = −0.46998	P = 0.6384
Ques8	b8 = 0.718713	z = 1.845764	P = 0.0649
Ques9	b9 = −0.083725	z = −0.147419	P = 0.8828
Ques10	b10 = 0.155926	z = 0.57686	P = 0.564

logit Y = −0.278368 −0.097036 Ques1 −0.515647 Ques2 +0.222503 Ques3 +0.670263 Ques4 +0.299508 Ques5 −0.373571 Ques6 −0.105121 Ques7 +0.718713 Ques8 −0.083725 Ques9 +0.155926 Ques10

Logistic regression – odds ratios

Parameter	Estimate	Odds Ratio	95% CI		
Constant	−0.278368				
Ques1	−0.097036	0.907524	0.290799	to	2.832189
Ques2	−0.515647	0.597114	0.238247	to	1.496538
Ques3	0.222503	1.2492	0.356246	to	4.380402
Ques4	0.670263	1.954751	0.48393	to	7.895871
Ques5	0.299508	1.349195	0.75798	to	2.401551
Ques6	−0.373571	0.688272	0.353693	to	1.33935
Ques7	−0.105121	0.900216	0.580708	to	1.395517
Ques8	0.718713	2.051791	0.956506	to	4.401272
Ques9	−0.083725	0.919684	0.302138	to	2.799442
Ques10	0.155926	1.16874	0.688076	to	1.985179

Logistic regression

Deviance goodness of fit chi-square =	34.595382	df = 48	P = 0.9267
Deviance (likelihood ratio) chi-square =	17.867511	df = 10	P = 0.0572
Intercept	b0 = −17.03837	z = −0.012798	P = 0.9898
Ques1	b1 = 0.969165	z = 0.953231	P = 0.3405
Ques2	b2 = −0.699573	z = −0.858767	P = 0.3905
Ques3	b3 = 2.080187	z = 1.818803	P = 0.0689
Ques4	b4 = 14.066614	z = 0.010566	P = 0.9916
Ques5	b5 = 0.662566	z = 0.991042	P = 0.3217
Ques6	b6 = −1.272351	z = −2.257605	P = 0.024
Ques7	b7 = −0.245328	z = −0.518584	P = 0.6041
Ques8	b8 = 0.447206	z = 0.634128	P = 0.526
Ques9	b9 = −0.602926	z = −0.565392	P = 0.5718
Ques10	b10 = 0.38782	z = 0.675565	P = 0.4993

logit Y = −17.03837 +0.969165 Ques1 −0.699573 Ques2 +2.080187 Ques3 +14.066614 Ques4
   +0.662566 Ques5 −1.272351 Ques6 −0.245328 Ques7 +0.447206 Ques8 −0.602926 Ques9
   +0.38782 Ques10

Logistic regression – odds ratios

Parameter	Estimate	Odds Ratio	95% CI	
Constant	−17.03837			
Ques1	0.969165	2.635742	0.359313	to 19.334482
Ques2	−0.699573	0.496797	0.10064	to 2.452386
Ques3	2.080187	8.005963	0.850911	to 75.325641
Ques4	14.066614	1285442.507217	* to *	
Ques5	0.662566	1.939764	0.523207	to 7.191577
Ques6	−1.272351	0.280172	0.092833	to 0.845569
Ques7	−0.245328	0.782448	0.309582	to 1.977586
Ques8	0.447206	1.563936	0.392578	to 6.230339
Ques9	−0.602926	0.547208	0.067677	to 4.424477
Ques10	0.38782	1.473765	0.478389	to 4.540208

Logistic regression

Deviance goodness of fit chi-square =	23.56364	df = 48	P = 0.9988
Deviance (likelihood ratio) chi-square =	13.666638	df = 10	P = 0.1887
Intercept	b0 = –33.753554	z = –0.009249	P = 0.9926
Ques1	b1 = 15.518733	z = 0.005601	P = 0.9955
Ques2	b2 = 15.884254	z = 0.006688	P = 0.9947
Ques3	b3 = –0.455762	z = –0.223705	P = 0.823
Ques4	b4 = –0.386598	z = –0.324645	P = 0.7454
Ques5	b5 = –0.705387	z = –1.181432	P = 0.2374
Ques6	b6 = –0.408138	z = –0.579483	P = 0.5623
Ques7	b7 = 0.751219	z = 1.362702	P = 0.173
Ques8	b8 = 1.225788	z = 1.723528	P = 0.0848
Ques9	b9 = –1.396153	z = –0.712108	P = 0.4764
Ques10	b10 = 0.308605	z = 0.44419	P = 0.6569

logit Y = –33.753554 +15.518733 Ques1 +15.884254 Ques2 –0.455762 Ques3 –0.386598 Ques4 –0.705387 Ques5 –0.408138 Ques6 +0.751219 Ques7 +1.225788 Ques8 –1.396153 Ques9 +0.308605 Ques10

Logistic regression – odds ratios

Parameter	Estimate	Odds Ratio	95% CI	
Constant	–33.753554			
Ques1	15.518733	5491613.021966	* to *	
Ques2	15.884254	7914867.440796	* to *	
Ques3	–0.455762	0.633965	0.011692 to	34.375165
Ques4	–0.386598	0.679364	0.065836 to	7.010381
Ques5	–0.705387	0.493917	0.153262 to	1.591745
Ques6	–0.408138	0.664887	0.1672 to	2.643995
Ques7	0.751219	2.119581	0.719461 to	6.244433
Ques8	1.225788	3.406848	0.845223 to	13.732018
Ques9	–1.396153	0.247547	0.005306 to	11.54829
Ques10	0.308605	1.361525	0.348856 to	5.313803

Logistic regression

Deviance goodness of fit chi-square =	67.926692	df = 48	P = 0.0306
Deviance (likelihood ratio) chi-square =	6.440918	df = 10	P = 0.777
Intercept	b0 = 0.560354	z = 0.630148	P = 0.5286
Ques1	b1 = −0.659849	z = −1.049261	P = 0.2941
Ques2	b2 = 0.333131	z = 0.715045	P = 0.4746
Ques3	b3 = 0.47504	z = 0.689311	P = 0.4906
Ques4	b4 = 0.158479	z = 0.235288	P = 0.814
Ques5	b5 = −0.017795	z = −0.058966	P = 0.953
Ques6	b6 = −0.157237	z = −0.43731	P = 0.6619
Ques7	b7 = 0.1225	z = 0.528747	P = 0.597
Ques8	b8 = 0.240712	z = 0.593525	P = 0.5528
Ques9	b9 = −0.775551	z = −1.282422	P = 0.1997
Ques10	b10 = 0.349784	z = 1.292479	P = 0.1962

logit Y = 0.560354 −0.659849 Ques1 +0.333131 Ques2 +0.47504 Ques3 +0.158479 Ques4
−0.017795 Ques5 −0.157237 Ques6 +0.1225 Ques7 +0.240712 Ques8 −0.775551 Ques9
+0.349784 Ques10

Logistic regression – odds ratios

Parameter	Estimate	Odds Ratio	95% CI		
Constant	0.560354				
Ques1	−0.659849	0.516929	0.150708	to	1.773073
Ques2	0.333131	1.39533	0.559902	to	3.477297
Ques3	0.47504	1.608078	0.416581	to	6.20747
Ques4	0.158479	1.171727	0.312966	to	4.386875
Ques5	−0.017795	0.982363	0.54375	to	1.774779
Ques6	−0.157237	0.854502	0.422338	to	1.728885
Ques7	0.1225	1.130319	0.717787	to	1.779944
Ques8	0.240712	1.272154	0.574545	to	2.816799
Ques9	−0.775551	0.46045	0.140739	to	1.506437
Ques10	0.349784	1.418761	0.834734	to	2.411406

Logistic regression

Deviance goodness of fit chi-square =	32.302568	df = 48	P = 0.9599
Deviance (likelihood ratio) chi-square =	8.348778	df = 10	P = 0.5948
Intercept	b0 = 17.06079	z = 0.01211	P = 0.9903
Ques1	b1 = 0.101337	z = 0.116365	P = 0.9074
Ques2	b2 = 0.037497	z = 0.047705	P = 0.962
Ques3	b3 = −0.40569	z = −0.351997	P = 0.7248
Ques4	b4 = −14.346333	z = −0.010183	P = 0.9919
Ques5	b5 = −0.946881	z = −1.553422	P = 0.1203
Ques6	b6 = 0.31155	z = 0.585036	P = 0.5585
Ques7	b7 = 0.411129	z = 1.078223	P = 0.2809
Ques8	b8 = −0.118517	z = −0.186559	P = 0.852
Ques9	b9 = −0.213207	z = −0.205365	P = 0.8373
Ques10	b10 = −0.239807	z = −0.506907	P = 0.6122

logit Y = 17.06079 +0.101337 Ques1 +0.037497 Ques2 −0.40569 Ques3 −14.346333 Ques4 −0.946881 Ques5 +0.31155 Ques6 +0.411129 Ques7 −0.118517 Ques8 −0.213207 Ques9 −0.239807 Ques10

Logistic regression – odds ratios

Parameter	Estimate	Odds Ratio	95% CI	
Constant	17.06079			
Ques1	0.101337	1.106649	0.200787 to	6.099354
Ques2	0.037497	1.038208	0.222453 to	4.845409
Ques3	−0.40569	0.666517	0.069626 to	6.380483
Ques4	−14.346333	5.88E−07	* to *	
Ques5	−0.946881	0.387949	0.11747 to	1.281211
Ques6	0.31155	1.36554	0.480854 to	3.877898
Ques7	0.411129	1.508521	0.714473 to	3.185054
Ques8	−0.118517	0.888237	0.255728 to	3.085169
Ques9	−0.213207	0.807989	0.105609 to	6.181706
Ques10	−0.239807	0.78678	0.311292 to	1.988561

Logistic regression

Deviance goodness of fit chi-square =	24.353285	df = 48	P = 0.9982
Deviance (likelihood ratio) chi-square =	6.891038	df = 10	P = 0.7357
Intercept	b0 = 16.270831	z = 0.011789	P = 0.9906
Ques1	b1 = −0.277624	z = −0.207555	P = 0.8356
Ques2	b2 = 0.863265	z = 1.221859	P = 0.2218
Ques3	b3 = 1.60163	z = 1.040112	P = 0.2983
Ques4	b4 = −13.946713	z = −0.010105	P = 0.9919
Ques5	b5 = −0.515653	z = −0.756623	P = 0.4493
Ques6	b6 = 0.398081	z = 0.626488	P = 0.531
Ques7	b7 = 0.486635	z = 0.993491	P = 0.3205
Ques8	b8 = −0.4272	z = −0.585172	P = 0.5584
Ques9	b9 = −0.988681	z = −0.889618	P = 0.3737
Ques10	b10 = −0.199107	z = −0.33003	P = 0.7414

logit Y = 16.270831 −0.277624 Ques1 +0.863265 Ques2 +1.60163 Ques3 −13.946713 Ques4 −0.515653 Ques5 +0.398081 Ques6 +0.486635 Ques7 −0.4272 Ques8 −0.988681 Ques9 −0.199107 Ques10

Logistic regression – odds ratios

Parameter	Estimate	Odds Ratio	95% CI		
Constant	16.270831				
Ques1	−0.277624	0.757582	0.055064	to	10.42294
Ques2	0.863265	2.37089	0.593639	to	9.468921
Ques3	1.60163	4.961111	0.242575	to	101.464025
Ques4	−13.946713	8.77E−07	*	to	*
Ques5	−0.515653	0.597111	0.157016	to	2.270725
Ques6	0.398081	1.488964	0.428565	to	5.173111
Ques7	0.486635	1.626833	0.622881	to	4.248944
Ques8	−0.4272	0.652333	0.155976	to	2.728233
Ques9	−0.988681	0.372067	0.042134	to	3.285547
Ques10	−0.199107	0.819463	0.251189	to	2.673365

Logistic regression

Deviance goodness of fit chi-square =	28.172444	df = 48	P = 0.99
Deviance (likelihood ratio) chi-square =	4.704105	df = 10	P = 0.91
Intercept	b0 = –17.881444	z = –0.012529	P = 0.99
Ques1	b1 = 0.282944	z = 0.241001	P = 0.8096
Ques2	b2 = 0.305274	z = 0.286027	P = 0.7749
Ques3	b3 = 0.634725	z = 0.520176	P = 0.6029
Ques4	b4 = 14.434372	z = 0.010113	P = 0.9919
Ques5	b5 = –0.049591	z = –0.086973	P = 0.9307
Ques6	b6 = 0.267743	z = 0.371971	P = 0.7099
Ques7	b7 = 0.349242	z = 0.815281	P = 0.4149
Ques8	b8 = –0.300718	z = –0.366824	P = 0.7138
Ques9	b9 = 0.200545	z = 0.189741	P = 0.8495
Ques10	b10 = –0.089891	z = –0.181108	P = 0.8563

logit Y = –17.881444 +0.282944 Ques1 +0.305274 Ques2 +0.634725 Ques3 +14.434372 Ques4 –0.049591 Ques5 +0.267743 Ques6 +0.349242 Ques7 –0.300718 Ques8 +0.200545 Ques9 –0.089891 Ques10

Logistic regression – odds ratios

Parameter	Estimate	Odds Ratio	95% CI	
Constant	–17.881444			
Ques1	0.282944	1.327031	0.132904 to	13.250245
Ques2	0.305274	1.356996	0.167533 to	10.991488
Ques3	0.634725	1.886503	0.172588 to	20.620753
Ques4	14.434372	1856813.190089	* to	*
Ques5	–0.049591	0.951618	0.311254 to	2.909447
Ques6	0.267743	1.307011	0.318851 to	5.357601
Ques7	0.349242	1.417992	0.612413 to	3.283244
Ques8	–0.300718	0.740286	0.148455 to	3.691521
Ques9	0.200545	1.222069	0.153966 to	9.6999
Ques10	–0.089891	0.914031	0.345524 to	2.417933

Logistic regression

Deviance goodness of fit chi-square =	69.542071	df = 48	P = 0.0227
Deviance (likelihood ratio) chi-square =	26.804505	df = 10	P = 0.0028
Intercept	$b0 = -1.437735$	$z = -1.424687$	P = 0.1542
Ques1	$b1 = -0.466126$	$z = -0.765742$	P = 0.4438
Ques2	$b2 = 0.009999$	$z = 0.020183$	P = 0.9839
Ques3	$b3 = 0.914307$	$z = 1.397987$	P = 0.1621
Ques4	$b4 = 0.751437$	$z = 0.92043$	P = 0.3573
Ques5	$b5 = -0.335735$	$z = -1.109215$	P = 0.2673
Ques6	$b6 = 0.536435$	$z = 1.345964$	P = 0.1783
Ques7	$b7 = -0.045903$	$z = -0.19093$	P = 0.8486
Ques8	$b8 = 0.461147$	$z = 1.191328$	P = 0.2335
Ques9	$b9 = 0.100562$	$z = 0.172729$	P = 0.8629
Ques10	$b10 = 0.104701$	$z = 0.359512$	P = 0.7192

logit Y = –1.437735 –0.466126 Ques1 +0.009999 Ques2 +0.914307 Ques3 +0.751437 Ques4 –0.335735 Ques5 +0.536435 Ques6 –0.045903 Ques7 +0.461147 Ques8 +0.100562 Ques9 +0.104701 Ques10

Logistic regression – odds ratios

Parameter	Estimate	Odds Ratio	95% CI	
Constant	–1.437735			
Ques1	–0.466126	0.627428	0.19029 to	2.068767
Ques2	0.009999	1.010049	0.382512 to	2.667107
Ques3	0.914307	2.495046	0.692434 to	8.990394
Ques4	0.751437	2.120044	0.427982 to	10.501813
Ques5	–0.335735	0.714812	0.394959 to	1.293696
Ques6	0.536435	1.709901	0.782931 to	3.734378
Ques7	–0.045903	0.955134	0.596237 to	1.530065
Ques8	0.461147	1.585892	0.742651 to	3.386586
Ques9	0.100562	1.105792	0.353271 to	3.461295
Ques10	0.104701	1.110378	0.627445 to	1.965019

Logistic regression

Deviance goodness of fit chi-square =	47.176607	df = 48	P = 0.5065
Deviance (likelihood ratio) chi-square =	10.511914	df = 10	P = 0.3968
Intercept	b0 = −2.142019	z = −1.760412	P = 0.0783
Ques1	b1 = −0.013462	z = −0.019002	P = 0.9848
Ques2	b2 = 0.982346	z = 1.26166	P = 0.2071
Ques3	b3 = 0.571674	z = 0.729405	P = 0.4658
Ques4	b4 = 0.190232	z = 0.229742	P = 0.8183
Ques5	b5 = −0.327255	z = −0.948243	P = 0.343
Ques6	b6 = −0.030992	z = −0.07203	P = 0.9426
Ques7	b7 = 0.308776	z = 1.109574	P = 0.2672
Ques8	b8 = 0.66784	z = 1.517188	P = 0.1292
Ques9	b9 = −1.048841	z = −1.386857	P = 0.1655
Ques10	b10 = −0.383393	z = −1.200702	P = 0.2299

logit Y = −2.142019 −0.013462 Ques1 +0.982346 Ques2 +0.571674 Ques3 +0.190232 Ques4 −0.327255 Ques5 −0.030992 Ques6 +0.308776 Ques7 +0.66784 Ques8 −1.048841 Ques9 −0.383393 Ques10

Logistic regression – odds ratios

Parameter	Estimate	Odds Ratio	95% CI		
Constant	−2.142019				
Ques1	−0.013462	0.986628	0.24611	to	3.955282
Ques2	0.982346	2.670716	0.580591	to	12.285289
Ques3	0.571674	1.77123	0.381191	to	8.230146
Ques4	0.190232	1.20953	0.238672	to	6.129608
Ques5	−0.327255	0.7209	0.366531	to	1.417879
Ques6	−0.030992	0.969484	0.417159	to	2.253095
Ques7	0.308776	1.361757	0.789268	to	2.349498
Ques8	0.66784	1.95002	0.822915	to	4.620863
Ques9	−1.048841	0.350343	0.079571	to	1.542531
Ques10	−0.383393	0.681545	0.364502	to	1.274352

Logistic regression

Deviance goodness of fit chi-square =	43.14225	df = 48	P = 0.6718
Deviance (likelihood ratio) chi-square =	12.367551	df = 10	P = 0.2612
Intercept	b0 = −0.632475	z = −0.602655	P = 0.5467
Ques1	b1 = −0.828645	z = −1.19654	P = 0.2315
Ques2	b2 = −0.339463	z = −0.557469	P = 0.5772
Ques3	b3 = 0.143166	z = 0.176952	P = 0.8595
Ques4	b4 = −0.557971	z = −0.667923	P = 0.5042
Ques5	b5 = 0.430477	z = 0.988039	P = 0.3231
Ques6	b6 = −0.308252	z = −0.660527	P = 0.5089
Ques7	b7 = −0.057619	z = −0.178559	P = 0.8583
Ques8	b8 = 0.659603	z = 1.407971	P = 0.1591
Ques9	b9 = 0.166703	z = 0.22457	P = 0.8223
Ques10	b10 = 0.29884	z = 0.739875	P = 0.4594

logit Y = −0.632475 −0.828645 Ques1 −0.339463 Ques2 +0.143166 Ques3 −0.557971 Ques4
    +0.430477 Ques5 −0.308252 Ques6 −0.057619 Ques7 +0.659603 Ques8 +0.166703 Ques9
    +0.29884 Ques10

Logistic regression – odds ratios

Parameter	Estimate	Odds Ratio	95% CI	
Constant	−0.632475			
Ques1	−0.828645	0.43664	0.112367 to	1.69672
Ques2	−0.339463	0.712152	0.215896 to	2.349097
Ques3	0.143166	1.153921	0.236319 to	5.63447
Ques4	−0.557971	0.572369	0.111327 to	2.942757
Ques5	0.430477	1.537991	0.65478 to	3.612536
Ques6	−0.308252	0.73473	0.294369 to	1.833847
Ques7	−0.057619	0.944009	0.501536 to	1.77685
Ques8	0.659603	1.934024	0.772135 to	4.844294
Ques9	0.166703	1.181404	0.275762 to	5.06131
Ques10	0.29884	1.348294	0.610913 to	2.975702

Logistic regression

Deviance goodness of fit chi-square =	66.358502	df = 48	P = 0.0406
Deviance (likelihood ratio) chi-square =	26.196768	df = 10	P = 0.0035
Intercept	b0 = −1.464145	z = −1.403351	P = 0.1605
Ques1	b1 = −0.274121	z = −0.445055	P = 0.6563
Ques2	b2 = 0.725411	z = 1.224624	P = 0.2207
Ques3	b3 = 0.001232	z = 0.001753	P = 0.9986
Ques4	b4 = 0.451171	z = 0.552508	P = 0.5806
Ques5	b5 = 0.312947	z = 0.934941	P = 0.3498
Ques6	b6 = −0.346155	z = −0.938036	P = 0.3482
Ques7	b7 = −0.036011	z = −0.144775	P = 0.8849
Ques8	b8 = 0.982558	z = 2.482547	P = 0.013
Ques9	b9 = −0.148679	z = −0.232405	P = 0.8162
Ques10	b10 = −0.534226	z = −1.870582	P = 0.0614

logit Y = −1.464145 −0.274121 Ques1 +0.725411 Ques2 +0.001232 Ques3 +0.451171 Ques4 +0.312947 Ques5 −0.346155 Ques6 −0.036011 Ques7 +0.982558 Ques8 −0.148679 Ques9 −0.534226 Ques10

Logistic regression – odds ratios

Parameter	Estimate	Odds Ratio	95% CI	
Constant	−1.464145			
Ques1	−0.274121	0.76024	0.227339	to 2.542306
Ques2	0.725411	2.06558	0.646888	to 6.595606
Ques3	0.001232	1.001233	0.252438	to 3.971147
Ques4	0.451171	1.57015	0.316856	to 7.780739
Ques5	0.312947	1.367449	0.709568	to 2.635289
Ques6	−0.346155	0.707403	0.343206	to 1.458069
Ques7	−0.036011	0.96463	0.59243	to 1.570669
Ques8	0.982558	2.67128	1.229775	to 5.802476
Ques9	−0.148679	0.861846	0.24597	to 3.019787
Ques10	−0.534226	0.586123	0.334881	to 1.025855

Logistic regression

Deviance goodness of fit chi-square =	68.15613	df = 48	P = 0.0294
Deviance (likelihood ratio) chi-square =	7.097097	df = 10	P = 0.7162
Intercept	b0 = −0.966166	z = −1.098367	P = 0.272
Ques1	b1 = 0.024229	z = 0.042166	P = 0.9664
Ques2	b2 = 0.504271	z = 1.05756	P = 0.2903
Ques3	b3 = −0.786974	z = −1.184402	P = 0.2363
Ques4	b4 = 0.336837	z = 0.498901	P = 0.6178
Ques5	b5 = 0.148792	z = 0.514297	P = 0.607
Ques6	b6 = 0.119305	z = 0.350283	P = 0.7261
Ques7	b7 = 0.136224	z = 0.612227	P = 0.5404
Ques8	b8 = 0.385936	z = 1.01254	P = 0.3113
Ques9	b9 = 0.394218	z = 0.677863	P = 0.4979
Ques10	b10 = −0.422266	z = −1.582391	P = 0.1136

logit Y = −0.966166 +0.024229 Ques1 +0.504271 Ques2 −0.786974 Ques3 +0.336837 Ques4 +0.148792 Ques5 +0.119305 Ques6 +0.136224 Ques7 +0.385936 Ques8 +0.394218 Ques9 −0.422266 Ques10

Logistic regression – odds ratios

Parameter	Estimate	Odds Ratio	95% CI		
Constant	−0.966166				
Ques1	0.024229	1.024525	0.332208	to	3.159624
Ques2	0.504271	1.655779	0.650321	to	4.215769
Ques3	−0.786974	0.45522	0.123778	to	1.674175
Ques4	0.336837	1.40051	0.372899	to	5.259943
Ques5	0.148792	1.160431	0.6582	to	2.045884
Ques6	0.119305	1.126713	0.577961	to	2.196486
Ques7	0.136224	1.145938	0.740908	to	1.772386
Ques8	0.385936	1.47099	0.696898	to	3.104918
Ques9	0.394218	1.483224	0.474441	to	4.636935
Ques10	−0.422266	0.655559	0.388567	to	1.106007

References

Abdullah, A.S.M., C.Y. Ming, C.K. Seng, C.Y. Ping, C.K. Fai, F.Y. Wing, H.W. Man, H.B. Kei, W.Y. Mun and W.M. Yee. 2003. "Effects of a brief sexual education intervention of the knowledge and attitudes of Chinese public school students". *Journal of HIV/AIDS Prevention & Education for Adolescents & Children* 5 (3–4): 129–49.

Agius, P.A., M.K. Pitts, A. Smith and A. Mitchell. 2010. "Sexual behaviour and related knowledge among a representative sample of secondary school students between 1997 and 2008". *Australian and New Zealand Journal of Public Health* 34 (5): 476–81.

Aggarwal, O., A.K. Sharma and P. Chhabra. 2000. "Study in sexuality of medical college students in India". *Journal of Adolescent Health* 26 (3): 226–29.

Agrawal, H.K., R.S. Rao, S. Chandrashekar and J.B. Coulter. 1999. "Knowledge of and attitudes to HIV/AIDS of senior secondary school pupils and trainee teachers in Udupi District, Karnataka, India". *Annals of Tropical Paediatrics* 19 (2): 143–49.

Ajzen, I. 1991. "The theory of planned behavior". *Organizational Behavior and Human Decision Processes* 50 (2): 211.

———. 2002. "Perceived behavioral control, self-efficacy, locus of control and the theory of planned behavior". *Journal of Applied Social Psychology* 32 (4): 665–83.

———. 2006. http://people.umass.edu/aizen/tpb.diag.html#null-link.

———. 2011. "The theory of planned behavior: Reactions and reflections". *Psychology & Health* 26 (9): 1113–27.

———. 2012. "The Theory of Planned Behavior". In *Handbook of theories of social psychology*, volume 1, edited by A.W. Kruglanski, P.A.M. Van Lange and E.T. Higgins. Thousand Oaks, CA: Sage Publications.

Al-Almaie, S.M. 2005. "Acquired immunodeficiency syndrome (AIDS) related knowledge and attitudes among male school students in Alkhobar, Saudi Arabia". *Journal of the Bahrain Medical Society* 17: 34–38.

Alene, G.D., J.G. Wheeler and H. Grosskurth. 2004. "Adolescent reproductive health and awareness of HIV among rural high school students, North Western Ethiopia". *AIDS Care* 16 (1): 57–68. doi: 10.1080/09540120310001633976.

Al-Iryani, B., Y.A. Raja'a, G. Kok and B. Van Den Borne. 2009. "HIV knowledge and stigmatization among adolescents in Yemeni schools". *International Quarterly of Community Health Education* 30 (4): 311–20.

Amoakoh-Coleman, M. 2006. "Knowledge, attitude and practices of STIs including HIV/AIDS among adolescents in Ghana". *Gender & Behaviour* 4 (2): 953–74.

Anderson, J.E., L. Kann, D. Holtzman, S. Arday, B. Truman and L. Kolbe. 1990. "HIV/AIDS knowledge and sexual behavior among high school students". *Family Planning Perspectives* 22 (6): 252–55.

Apinundecha, C., W. Laohasiriwong, M.P. Cameron and S. Lim. 2007. "A community participation intervention to reduce HIV/AIDS stigma, Nakhon Ratchasima Province, Northeast Thailand". *AIDS Care* 19 (9): 1157–65.

Archibald, C. 2007. "Knowledge and attitudes toward HIV/AIDS and risky sexual behaviors among Caribbean African American female adolescents". *Journal of the Association of Nurses in AIDS Care* 18 (4): 64–72.

Armitage, C.J., and M. Conner. 2001. "Efficacy of the theory of planned behavior: A meta-analytic review". *British Journal of Social Psychology* 40: 471–99.

Babbie, E. 1995. *The Practice of Social Research* (seventh edition). Belmont, CA: Wadsworth Publishing Company.

Bankole, A., A. Biddlecom, G. Guiella, S. Singh and E. Zulu. 2007. "Sexual behavior, knowledge and information sources of very young adolescents in four Sub-Saharan African Countries". *African Journal of Reproductive Health* 11 (3): 28–43.

Barss, P., M. Grivna, M. Ganczak, R. Bernsen, F. Al-Maskari, H.E. Agab, F. Al-Awadhi, H. Al-Baloushi, S. Al-Dhaheri, J. Al-Dhahri, A. Al-Jaberi, S. Al-Kaabi, A. Khouri, H. Al-Kitbi, D. Al-Mansoori, M. Al-Marzouqi, S. Al-Muhairy, W. Al-Neaimi, E. Al-Shamsi, A.M. Zahmi and A. Yammahi. 2009. "Effects of a rapid peer-based HIV/AIDS educational intervention on knowledge and attitudes of high school students in a high-income Arab country". *Journal of Acquired Immune Deficiency Syndromes* 52 (1): 86–98.

Becker, M.H., D.P. Haefner, S.V. Kasl, J.P. Kihscht, L.A. Maiman and I.M. Rosenstock. 1997. "Selected psychosocial models and correlates of individual health-related behaviors". *Medical Care* 15 (5): 27–46.

Bertolli, J., A.D. McNaghten, M. Campsmith, L.M. Lee, R. Leman, R.T. Bryan and J.W. Buehler. 2004. "Surveillance systems monitoring HIV/AIDS and HIV risk behaviors among American Indians and Alaska Natives". *AIDS Education and Prevention* 16 (3): 218–37.

Bhalla, S., H. Chandwani, D. Singh, C. Somasundaram, S.K. Rasania and S. Singh. 2005. "Knowledge about HIV/AIDS among senior secondary school students in Jamnagar, Gujarat". *Health and Population Perspectives and Issues* 28 (4): 178–88.

Bhowon, U., and J. Ah-Kion. 2005. "AIDS/HIV: Low prevalence, moderate knowledge and liberal attitudes – a study of youths in Mauritius". *Journal of Psychology in Africa: South of the Sahara, the Caribbean and Afro-Latin America* 15 (1): 25–30.

Borire, A.A., O.A. Oyekunle, T. Izekor, A. Akinlonu, A.O. Okanlawon and C.C. Noronha. 2008. "Comparing the knowledge and attitude about HIV/AIDS and the sexual behaviour of secondary school students of a missionary school and a public school". *Nigerian Quarterly Journal of Hospital Medicine* 18 (4): 206–10.

Breault, A.J., and E.C. Polifroni. 1992. "Caring for people with AIDS: Nurses' attitudes and feelings". *Journal of Advanced Nursing* 17 (1): 21–27.

Bureau of Statistics. 2002. *2002 Population and Housing Census: Guyana National Report*. http://www.statisticsguyana.gov.gy/census.html.

Buseh, A.G., C.G. Park, P.E. Stevens, B.J. McElmurry and S.T. Kelber. 2006. "HIV/AIDS stigmatizing attitudes among young people in Swaziland: Individual and environmental factors". *Journal of HIV/AIDS Prevention in Children & Youth* 7 (1): 97–120.

Cai, Y., H. Hong, R. Shi, X. Ye, G. Xu, S. Li and L. Shen. 2008. "Long-term follow-up study on peer-led school-based HIV/AIDS prevention among youths in Shanghai". *International Journal of STD & AIDS* 19 (12): 848–50.

Camara, B., R. Lee, J. Gatwood, H.-U. Wagner, R. Cazal-Gamelsy and E. Boisson. 2003. "The Caribbean HIV/AIDS epidemic epidemiological status/success stories: A summary". *CAREC Surveillance Report* 23: 1–16.

Cheng, Y., C.H. Lou, L.M. Mueller, S.L. Zhao, J.H. Yang, X.W. Tu and E.S. Gao. 2008. "Effectiveness of a school-based AIDS education program among rural students in HIV high epidemic area of China". *Journal of Adolescent Health* 42 (2): 184–91.

Curran, J.W., H.W. Jaffe, A.M. Hardy, W.M. Morgan, R.M. Selik and T.J. Dondero. 1988. "Epidemiology of HIV Infection and AIDS in the United States". *Science* 239: 610–16.

Currie, C., O. Samdal, W. Boyce and R. Smith. 2001. *Health behaviour in school-aged children: A WHO cross-national study: Research protocol for the 2001/2002 survey*. Copenhagen: WHO.

Dias, S.F., M.G. Matos and A.C. Alves. 2006. "AIDS-related stigma and attitudes towards AIDS-infected people among adolescents". *AIDS Care* 18 (3): 208–14.

DiClemente, R.J., C.B. Boyer and S. Mills. 1987. "Prevention of AIDS among adolescents: Strategies for the development of comprehensive risk-reduction health education programs". *Health Education Research* 2: 287–91.

DiClemente, R.J., C.B. Boyer and E.S. Morales. 1988. "Minorities and AIDS: Knowledge, attitudes and misconceptions among black and Latino adolescents". *American Journal of Public Health* 78 (1): 55–57.

DiClemente, R.J., J. Zorn and L. Temoshok. 1986. "Adolescents and AIDS: A survey of knowledge, attitudes and beliefs about AIDS in San Francisco". *American Journal of Public Health* 76: 1443–45.

———. 1987. "The association of gender, ethnicity and length of residence in the Bay Area to adolescents' knowledge and attitudes about acquired immune deficiency syndrome". *Journal of Applied Social Psychology* 17 (3): 216–30.

Dumitrescu, A.L., W. Wagle, B.C. Dogaru and B. Manolescu. 2011. "Modeling the theory of planned behavior for intention to improve oral health behaviors: the impact of attitudes, knowledge, and current behavior". *Journal of Oral Science* 53 (3): 369–77.

El-Gadi, S., A. Abudher and M. Sammud. 2008. "HIV-related knowledge and stigma among high school students in Libya". *International Journal of STD & AIDS* 19 (3): 178–83.

Esiet, A.O., U. Esiet, S. Philliber and W.W. Philliber. *2009.* "Changes in knowledge and attitudes among junior secondary students exposed to the family life and HIV education curriculum in Lagos State, Nigeria". African Journal of Reproductive Health 13 (3): 37–46.

Fisher, J.D., and W.A. Fisher. 1992. "Changing AIDS risk behaviour". *Psychological Bulletin* 111: 455–74.

Francis, S.A., W.K. Lam, J.D. Cance and V.K. Hogan. 2009. "What's the 411? Assessing the feasibility of providing African American adolescents with HIV/AIDS prevention education in a faith-based setting". *Journal of Religion & Health* 48 (2): 164–77.

Francis, S.A., and J. Liverpool. 2009. "A review of faith-based HIV prevention programs". *Journal of Religion & Health* 48: 6–15.

Genrich, G.L., and B.A. Brathwaite. 2005. "Response of religious groups to HIV/AIDS as a sexually transmitted infection in Trinidad". *BMC Public Health* 5: 121. doi:10.1186/1471-2458-5-121.

Glenn, B.L., and K.P. Wilson. 2008. "African American adolescent perceptions of vulnerability and resilience to HIV". *Journal Transcultural Nursing* 19 (3): 259–65.

Goodman, E., and A.T. Cohall. 1989. "Acquired immunodeficiency syndrome and adolescents: knowledge, attitudes, beliefs and behaviors in a New York City adolescent minority population". *Pediatrics* 84 (1): 36–42.

Gordon, D.E., L.R. Ghazaryan, J. Maslak, B.J. Anderson, K.S. Brousseau, A.F. Carrascal and L.C. Smith. 2012. "Projections of diagnosed HIV infection in children and adolescents in New York State". *Paediatric and Perinatal Epidemiology* 26 (2): 131–39.

Griffith, D.M., B. Campbell, J.O. Allen, K.J. Robinson and S. Kretman. 2010. "Your Blessed Health: An HIV prevention program bridging public health and faith communities. *Public Health Reports* 125 (1): 4–11.

Grunseit, A. 1997. *Impact of HIV and Sexual Health Education on the Sexual Behaviour of Young People: A Review Update.* Geneva: Joint United Nations Programme on HIV/AIDS. http://data.unaids.org/Publications/IRC-pub01/jc010-impactyoungpeople_en.pdf.

Halcon, L., T. Beuhring and R.W. Blum. 2000. *A portrait of adolescent health in the Caribbean 2000.* Minneapolis, MN: WHO Collaborating Centre on Adolescent Health, University of Minnesota and PAHO.

Hancock, T., B.I. Mikhail, A. Santos, A. Nguyen, H. Nguyen and D. Bright. 1999. "A comparison of HIV/AIDS knowledge among high school freshmen and senior students". *Journal of Community Health Nursing* 16 (3): 151–63.

Herek, G.M., J.P. Capitanio and K.F. Widaman. 2002. "HIV-related stigma and knowledge in the United States: Prevalence and trends, 1991–1999". *American Journal of Public Health* 92 (3): 371–77.

Hermes, G. (2001). *Press Conference by Joint United Nations Programme on HIV/AIDS (UNAIDS).* Georgetown, Guyana.

HIV and the Workplace. (2000). Georgetown, Guyana: National AIDS Programme Secretariat (NAPS), Ministry of Health.

Holtzman, D., R. Lowry, L. Kann, J.L. Collins and L.J. Kolbe. 1994. "Changes in HIV-related information sources, instruction, knowledge and behaviors among US high school students, 1989 and 1990". *American Journal of Public Health* 84 (3): 388–93.

Huang, H., X. Ye, Y. Cai, L. Shen, G. Xu, R. Shi and X. Jin. 2008. "Study on peer-led school-based HIV/AIDS prevention among youths in a medium-sized city in China". *International Journal of STD & AIDS* 19 (5): 342–46.

Huskinson, T.L.H., and G. Haddock. 2004. "Assessing individual differences in attitude structure: Variance in the chronic reliance of affective and cognitive information". *Journal of Experimental Social Psychology* 40 (1): 82–90.

Imperato, M.A. 1996. "Acquired immunodeficiency syndrome and suburban adolescents: Knowledge, attitudes, behaviors and risks". *Journal of Community Health* 21: 329–47.

Inciardi, J.A., J.L. Syvertsen and H.L. Surratt. 2005. "HIV/AIDS in the Caribbean Basin". *AIDS Care: Psychological and Socio-medical Aspects of AIDS/HIV* 17 (S1): 9–25.

Kelly, M.J., and B. Bain. 2004. *Education and HIV/AIDS in the Caribbean.* Kingston: Ian Randle Publishers.

Kennedy, B.R., and C.C. Jenkins. 2011. "Promoting African American women and sexual assertiveness in reducing HIV/AIDS: An analytical review of the research literature". *Journal of Cultural Diversity* 18 (4): 142–49.

Lahai-Momoh, J.C., and M.W. Ross. 1997. "HIV/AIDS Prevention-Related Social Skills and Knowledge among Adolescents in Sierra Leone, West Africa". *African Journal of Reproductive Health/La Revue Africaine de la Santé Reproductive* 1 (1): 37–44.

Lau, J.T.F., H.Y. Tsui and K. Chan. 2005. "Reducing discriminatory attitudes toward people living with HIV/AIDS (PLWHA) in Hong Kong: An intervention study using an integrated knowledge-based PLWHA participation and cognitive approach". *AIDS Care* 17 (1): 85–101.

Lindley, L.L., J.D. Coleman, B.W. Gaddist and J. White. 2010. "Informing faith-based HIV/AIDS interventions: HIV-related knowledge and stigmatizing attitudes at Project F.A.I.T.H. churches in South Carolina". *Public Health Reports* 125 (1): 12–20.

Li, S., H. Huang, Y. Cai, X. Ye, X. Shen, R. Shi and G. Xu. 2010. "Evaluation of a school-based HIV/AIDS peer-led prevention programme: The first intervention trial for children of migrant workers in China". *International Journal of STD & AIDS* 21: 82–86.

Liverpool, J., M. McGhee, C. Lollis, M. Beckford and D. Levine. 2002. "Knowledge, attitudes and behavior of homeless African American adolescents: Implications for HIV/AIDS prevention". *Journal of the National Medical Association* 94 (4): 257–63.

Macchi, M.L., L.S. Benítez, A. Corvalán, C. Nuñez and D. Ortigoza. 2008. "Knowledge, attitudes and behavior related to HIV/AIDS in high-school aged youth in the metropolitan area of Asuncion, Paraguay". *Revista de la Sociedad Boliviana de Pediatría* 47 (3): 188–99.

Mahat, G., and M.A. Scoloveno. 2006. "HIV/AIDS knowledge, attitudes and beliefs among Nepalese adolescents". *Journal of Advanced Nursing* 53 (5): 583–90.

Manji, A., R. Pena and R. Dubrow. 2007. "Sex, condoms, gender roles and HIV transmission knowledge among adolescents in Leon, Nicaragua: Implications for HIV prevention". *AIDS Care* 19 (8): 989–95.

Matos, M., and S. Aventura. 2003. *A sau´de dos adolescents Portugueses (quatro anos depois)*. Lisboa: FMH.

McManus, A., and L. Dhar. 2008. "Study of knowledge, perception and attitude of adolescent girls towards STIs/HIV, safer sex and sex education: A cross sectional survey of urban adolescent school girls in South Delhi, India". *BMC Women's Health* 8: 12. doi:10.1186/1472-6874-8-12.

Meng, X., A.F. Anderson, L. Wang, Z. Li, W. Guo, Z. Lee, H. Jin and Y. Cai. 2010. "An exploratory survey of money boys and HIV transmission risk in Jilin Province, PR China". *AIDS Research and Therapy* 7: 17. doi:10.1186/1742-6405-7-17.

Ministry of Health. 2008. *Guyana Behavioural Surveillance Survey 2008/2009 Report.* Georgetown, Guyana: Ministry of Health, National AIDS Programme Secretariat.

Movahed, M., and S. Shoaa. 2010. "On attitude towards HIV/AIDS among Iranian students (case study: high school students in Shiraz City)". *Pakistan Journal of Biological Sciences* 13 (6): 271–78.

Mushi, D.L., R.M. Mpembeni and A. Jahn. 2007. "Knowledge about safe motherhood and HIV/AIDS among school pupils in a rural area in Tanzania". *BMC Pregnancy and Childbirth* 7: 5. doi: 10.1186/1471-2393-7-5.

National Institutes of Health. 1997. *Interventions to Prevent HIV Risk Behavior.* Washington, DC: National Institutes of Health.

Noden, B.H., A. Gomes and A. Ferreira. 2010. "Influence of religious affiliation and education on HIV knowledge and HIV-related sexual behaviors among unmarried youth in rural central Mozambique". *AIDS Care* 22 (10): 1285–94.

Nodin, N., S. Moreira and A.M. Ourô. 2004. "Portugal". In *International Encyclopedia of Sexuality*, edited by R.T. Francoeur and R.J. Noonan, 502–46. New York: Continuum International Publishing Group.

Norman, L., R. Carr and J. Jiménez. 2006. "Sexual stigma and sympathy: Attitudes toward persons living with HIV in Jamaica". *Culture, Health & Sexuality* 8 (5): 423–33. doi: 10.1080/13691050600855748.

Nwokocha, A.R.C., and B.A.N Nwakoby. 2002. "Knowledge, attitude and behavior of secondary (high) school students concerning HIV/AIDS in Enugu, Nigeria, in the year 2000". *Journal of Pediatric and Adolescent Gynecology* 15 (2): 93–96.

Odu, O.O., A. Olarinmoye, J.O. Bamidele, B.E. Egbewale, O.A. Amusan and A.O. Olowu. 2008. "Knowledge, attitudes to HIV/AIDS and sexual behaviour of students in a tertiary institution in south-western Nigeria". *The European Journal of Contraception and Reproductive Health Care* 13 (1): 90–96.

Odusanya, O.K. and O.M. Bankole. 2006. "A survey of information sources used by secondary school students in Ogun State, Nigeria for knowledge and attitudes towards HIV/AIDS". *African Journal of Library, Archives and Information Science* 16 (1): 53–63.

PAHO. 2003. *PAHO prepared to help Caribbean reduce high cervical cancer rate.* Press release. www.paho.org/English/DD/PIN/pr031211.htm.

———. 2003. Gender and HIV/AIDS [Fact Sheet]. Washington, DC: Author.

Pattullo, A.L., M. Malonza, G.G. Kimani, A. Muthee, P.A. Otieno, K. Odhiambo, S. Moses and F.A. Plummer. 1994. "Survey of knowledge, behaviour and attitudes relating to HIV infection and AIDS among Kenyan secondary school students". *AIDS Care* 6 (2): 173–81.

Pramanik, S., M. Chartier and C. Koopman. 2006. "HIV/AIDS stigma and knowledge among predominantly middle-class high school students in New Delhi, India". *Journal of Communicable Diseases* 38 (1): 57–69.

Robillard, H.H. 2001. "The Jamaican adolescent: An assessment of knowledge and attitudes regarding HIV/AIDS". *Pediatric Nursing* 27 (2): 176–79.

Rondini, S., and J.K. Krugu. 2009. "Knowledge, attitude and practices study on reproductive health among secondary school students in Bolgatanga, Upper East Region, Ghana". *African Journal of Reproductive Health* 13 (4): 51–66.

Rossem, R.V., H. Berten and C.V. Tuyckom. 2010. "AIDS knowledge and sexual activity among Flemish secondary school students: A multilevel analysis of the effects of type of education". *BMC Public Health* 10: 30. doi:10.1186/1471-2458-10-30.

Sallar, A.M. 2009. "Correlates of misperceptions in HIV knowledge and attitude towards people living with HIV/AIDS (PLWHAs) among in-school and out-of-school adolescents in Ghana". *African Health Sciences* 9 (2): 82–91.

Savaser, S. 2003. "Knowledge and attitudes of high school students about AIDS: A Turkish perspective". *Public Health Nursing* 20 (1): 72–79.

Sechrist, W. 1997. "Personalizing HIV infection: Moving students closer to believing 'this could actually happen to me'!" *Journal of HIV/AIDS Prevention & Education for Adolescents and Children* 1: 105–07.

Shen, L.X., H. Hong, Y. Cai, X.M. Jin and R. Shi. 2008. "Effectiveness of peer education in HIV/STD prevention at different types of senior high schools in Shanghai, People's Republic of China". *International Journal of STD & AIDS* 19 (11): 761–67.

Smith, K.W., S.A. McGraw, S.L. Crawford, L.A. Costa and J.B. McKinlay. 1993. "HIV risk among Latino adolescents in two New England cities". *American Journal of Public Health* 83 (10): 1395–99.

Stall, R.D., T.J. Coates and C. Hoff. 1988. "Changes in sexual behavior among gay and bisexual men: Responses to the threat of AIDS". *American Psychologist* 43 (11): 878–85.

Stigler, M.H., K.C. Kugler, K.A. Komro, M.T. Leshabari and K.I. Klepp. 2006. "AIDS education for Tanzanian youth: A mediation analysis". *Health Education Research* 21 (4): 441–51.

Sullivan, S.G., X. Jie, F. Yuji, S. Su, X. Chen, D. Xinping, G. Yun, D. Zhi, W. Zunyou and China CIPRA Project 2 Team. 2010. "Stigmatizing attitudes and behaviors toward PLHIV in rural China". *AIDS Care* 22 (1): 104–11.

Swenson, R.R., C.J Rizzo, L.K. Brown, N. Payne, R.J. DiClemente, L.F. Salazar, P.A. Venable, M.P. Carey, R.F. Valois, D. Romer and M. Hennessy. 2009. "Prevalence and correlates of HIV testing among sexually active African American adolescents in 4 US cities". *Sexually Transmitted Diseases* 36 (9): 584–91.

Tavoosi, A., A. Zaferani, A. Enzevaei, P. Tajik and Z. Ahmadinezhad. 2004. "Knowledge and attitude towards HIV/AIDS among Iranian students". *BMC Public Health* 4: 17.

Tebourski, F., and D.B. Alaya. 2004. "Knowledge and attitudes of high school students regarding HIV/AIDS in Tunisia: Does more knowledge lead to more positive attitudes?" *Journal of Adolescent Health* 34 (3): 161–62.

The Republic of Guyana: The Census Road. 2002. Georgetown: Guyana Population and Housing Census.

Toure, B., K. Koffi, V. Kouassi-Gohou, E. Kokoun, O. Angbo-Effi, N.M. Koffi and A.J. Diarra-Nam. 2005. "Awareness, attitudes and practices of secondary school students in relation to HIV/AIDS in Abidjan, Ivory Coast". *Medecine Tropicale* 65 (4): 346–48.

Trinitapoli, J. 2009. "Religious teachings and influences on the ABCs of HIV prevention in Malawi". *Social Science & Medicine* 69 (2): 199–209.

UNAIDS. 2008. *Epidemiological Fact Sheet on HIV and AIDS, 2008 Update.* Geneva, Switzerland: World Health Organization.

———. 2008. *Regions & countries: HIV and AIDS estimates.* Geneva, Switzerland.

———. 2009. *AIDS Epidemic Update.* 37. Geneva, Switzerland.

———. 2010. *Narrative Report-Turkey.* Geneva, Switzerland.

———. 2010. *The status of HIV in the Caribbean.* Port of Spain, Trinidad and Tobago: UNAIDS Caribbean Regional Support Team,

———. 2010. *Report on the global AIDS epidemic.* Geneva, Switzerland.

———. 2011. "2,500 young people newly infected with HIV every day, according to Opportunity in Crisis". Feature Story, Geneva, Switzerland: UNAIDS

UNAIDS/WHO. 2004. *Islamic Republic of Iran: Epidemiological fact sheet on HIV/AIDS and sexually transmitted infections.* Geneva: UNAIDS/WHO. http://data.unaids.org/publications/Fact-Sheets01/iran_en.pdf.

UNGASS. 2004, 2006, 2008. *UNGASS Reports: Antigua and Barbuda, Bahamas, Barbados, Belize, Cuba, Dominica, Dominican Republic, Grenada, Guyana, Haiti, Jamaica, St Kitts and Nevis, St Lucia, St Vincent and the Grenadines, Suriname, and Trinidad and Tobago.*

———. 2009. *Guyana Country Progress Report*

———. 2010. *Guyana Country Progress Report.*

Uutela, A. 1976. "Asenteet ja ulkoinen käyttäytyminen: historiallinen katsaus asennetutkimuksen syntyyn, asenteen neobehavioristisen ja kvasifenomenologisen mallin jäljitys sekä 'asenne – ulkoinen käyttäytyminen' – ongelman tarkastelu mainittujen mallien avulla erityisesti mittausteknisessä kirjallisuudessa". *Research Reports.* Department of Social Psychology, University of Helsinki.

Välimäki, M., T. Suominen and I. Peate. 1998. "Attitudes of professionals, students and the general public to HIV/AIDS and people with HIV/AIDS: A review of the research". *Journal of Advanced Nursing* 27 (4): 752–59.

Wagbatsoma, V.A., and O.H. Okojie. *2006.* "Knowledge of HIV/AIDS and sexual practices among adolescents in Benin City Nigeria". *African Journal of Reproductive Health* 10 (3): 76–83.

Walker, H.S. 1992. "Teenagers' knowledge of the acquired immunodeficiency syndrome and associated risk behaviors". *Journal of Pediatric Nursing* 7: 246–50.

Walusimbi, M., and J.G. Okonsky. 2004. "Knowledge and attitude of nurses caring for patients with HIV/AIDS in Uganda". *Applied Nursing Research* 17 (2): 92–99.

World Bank. 2011. *World Development Indicators.*

Wu, Z., S.G. Sullivan, Y. Wang, M.J. Rotheram-Borus and R. Detels. 2007. "Evolution of China's response to HIV/AIDS". *Lancet* 369 (9562): 679–90.

Yazdi, C.A., K. Aschbacher, A. Arvantaj, H.M. Naser, E. Abdollahi, A. Asadi, M. Mousavi, M.R. Narmani, M. Kianpishe, F. Nicfallah and A.K. Moghadam. 2006. "Knowledge, attitudes and sources of information regarding HIV/AIDS in Iranian adolescents". *AIDS Care* 18 (8): 1004–10.

Ye, X.X., H. Huang, S.H. Li, G. Xu, Y. Cai, T. Chen, L.X. Shen and R. Shi. 2009. "HIV/AIDS education effects on behaviour among senior high school students in a medium-sized city in China". *International Journal of STD & AIDS* 20 (8): 549–52.

Yoo, H., S.H. Lee, B.E. Kwon, S. Chung and S. Kim. 2005. "HIV/AIDS knowledge, attitudes, related behaviors and sources of information among Korean adolescents". *The Journal of School Health* 75 (10): 393–99.

Zuckerman, P., ed. 2000. *Du Bois on religion.* Walnut Creek, CA: AltaMira Press. www.aids.gov.hk

Recommended Further Reading

Balabanova, Y., R. Coker, R.A. Atun, and F. Drobniewski. 2006. "Stigma and HIV infection in Russia." *AIDS Care* 18 (7): 846–52.

Bandura, A. 1994. "Social cognitive theory and exercise of control over HIV infection". In *Preventing AIDS: Theories and methods of behavioral interventions*, edited by R.J. DiClemente and J.L. Peterson, 25–29. New York: Plenum.

Centers for Disease Control and Prevention. 1993. "U.S. AIDS cases reported through June 1993". *HIV/AIDS Surveillance Report* 5 (2): 2–19.

Education Development Center. 2005. *HHD and UNESCO to advance the education sector's response to HIV/AIDS in the Caribbean*. Waltham, MA: Education Development Center.

Fishbein, M. 1997. "Theoretical models of HIV prevention". In *Interventions to Prevent HIV Risk Behaviors, Programs and Abstracts*. NIH Consensus Development Conference. Bethesda, MD: NIH.

Fishbein, M., and M. Guinan. 1996. "Behavioral science and public health: A necessary partnership for HIV prevention". *Public Health Reports* 3: 5–10.

Fishbein, M., S.E. Middlestadt, and P.J. Hitchcock. 1991. "Using information to change sexually transmitted disease-related behavior: An analysis based on the theory of reasoned action". In *Research issues in human behavior and sexually transmitted disease in the AIDS era*, edited by J.N. Wasserheit, S.O. Arol and K.K. Holmes, 243–57. Washington, DC: American Society for Microbiology.

Goodwin, R., A. Kozlova, G. Nizharadze and G. Polyakova. 2004. "High-risk behaviors and beliefs and knowledge about HIV transmission among school and shelter children in Eastern Europe". *Sexually Transmitted Diseases* 31(11): 670–75.

Hospers, H.J., and G. Kok. 1995. "Determinants of safe and risk-taking sexual behavior among gay men: A review". *AIDS Education and Prevention* 7 (1): 74–94.

Kelly, J.A., D.A. Murphy, K.J. Sikkema and S.C. Kalichman. 1993. "Psychological interventions to prevent HIV infection are urgently needed: New priorities for behavioral research in the second decade of AIDS". *American Psychologist* 48 (10): 1023–34.

Liu, H., Z. Hu, X. Li, B. Stanton, S. Naar-King and H. Yang. 2006.
"Understanding interrelationships among HIV-related stigma, concern
about HIV infection and intent to disclose HIV serostatus: A pretest-
posttest study in a rural area of eastern China". *AIDS Patient Care & STDs*
20 (2): 133–42.

Mbanya, D.N., R. Zebaze, A.P. Kengne, E.M. Minkoulou and P.B. Awah.
2001. "Knowledge, attitudes and practices of nursing staff in a rural
hospital of Cameroon: How much does the health care provider know
about the human immunodeficiency virus/acquired immune deficiency
syndrome"? *International Nursing Review* 48 (4): 241–49.

Qu, B., Y. Zhang, G. Haiqiang and G. Sun. 2010. "Relationship between
HIV/AIDS Knowledge and Attitude among Student Nurses: A Structural
Equation Model". *Aids Patient Care and STDs* 24 (1): 59–63.

Ralph J. DiClemente Center for AIDS Prevention Studies. 1992.
"Epidemiology of AIDS, HIV prevalence and HIV incidence among
adolescents". *Journal of School Health* 62 (7): 325–30.

Rosenstock, I.M., V.J. Strecher and M.H. Becker. 1994. "The health belief
model and HIV risk behavior change". In *Preventing AIDS: Theories and
methods of behavioral interventions*, edited by R.J. DiClemente and J. L.
Peterseon, 5–24. New York: Plenum.

Serlo, K., and H. Aavarinne. 1999. "Attitudes of university students towards
HIV/AIDS". *Journal of Advanced Nursing* 29 (2): 463–70.

Turner, C.F., H.G. Miller and L.E. Moses. 1989. *AIDS sexual behavior and
intravenous drug use*. Washington, DC: National Academy Press.

Visser, M.J., J.D. Makin and K. Lehobye. 2006. "Stigmatizing attitudes of
the community towards people living with HIV/AIDS". *Journal of
Community & Applied Social Psychology* 16 (1): 42–58.

Index

CPSIA information can be obtained at www.ICGtesting.com
Printed in the USA
BVOW02s0336190214

345345BV00004B/10/P